In this book, Katherine has gifted expectant mothers with a hopeful and encouraging perspective on their journey through pregnancy, childbirth, and the postpartum period: You are chosen by God for the high and holy calling of participating in His ongoing work of creation in the world. Thanks, Katherine, for this reminder of the sacredness of pregnancy and childbirth, and for your practical suggestions on how to savour this truth during the sometimes uncomfortable realities of pregnancy and childbirth.

> ----Dr. Carolyn Watts, obstetrician and spiritual director

Chosen provides a much needed Christian voice in the world of pregnancy and birth. It is rare to see a birth professional (Katherine is a doula) speak to labor through a biblical lens, providing encouragement and true empowerment in a season often riddled with anxiety. I would recommend this book for any expecting woman to prepare her mind and heart to meet her baby.

> -----Phylicia Masonheimer, author of *Stop Calling Me Beautiful* and host of the *Verity* podcast

There is such tangled information in the world in regards to birth, postpartum, and even the loss of a child. This book is a refreshing Biblical approach that many women of childbearing age will be blessed by as they read through it.

> ----Callie Domingues, Founder & Managing Director of GROUNDED Ministry & Conferences, and Blogger at *Mama's Coffee Shop*

This beautiful book is a reminder to all mothers that God has chosen them for the task of growing, birthing, and raising their precious children. We are reminded of God's incredible design for pregnancy and encouraged to release fears and anxiety and lean into His presence and peace. He created us to do this! This book is a great resource for women who want to grow closer to God and their babies during pregnancy. Each birth is as unique as the woman doing the birthing, and this is a book every pregnant mom needs to read, no matter what her birth plan looks like.

> ----Stephanie Thurling, mom of 3 + co-founder of *Raising Prayerful Kids*

Katherine has created a beautiful resource, encouraging mothers to abide in Christ with peace and trust as they co-create with Him. Pregnancy, birth, and motherhood can be transformative, worshipful experiences that draw us more into God; Katherine takes you along with her doula heart and shows you how.

  ----Aubry G. Smith, childbirth educator, birth doula & author of *Holy Labor: How Childbirth Shapes a Woman's Soul*

At a time when there can be far too much confusion, a lack of education and information, and therefore fear surrounding childbirth for many mamas, Katherine Newsom seeks to fill the void in her beautiful new book, 'Chosen'. This wonderful resource will provide the encouragement, knowledge, wisdom, and gospel-centered perspective you will need as you walk along the journey of childbearing. I highly recommend it!

  ----Rebekah Hargraves, Author of *Lies Moms Believe: And How the Gospel Refutes Them*, and host of the *Hargraves Home & Hearth* podcast

I am pregnant with my second child and I was thrilled to find Katherine's [podcast] *Chosen: Birth + Faith Through a Doula Lens*. I found this [podcast] to be a tender reminder of God's design and intent for this unique season of life. Katherine finds a way to interweave truth from Scripture with birth affirmations, which spurs mothers on in their pregnancy/birth journey. If you are pregnant and have been eager to see this special time in life through a bibilical lens, this is [the podcast] for you!

  ----Jessica Schatzle, blogger at *www.thesesoulstirrings.blogspot.com*

Chosen

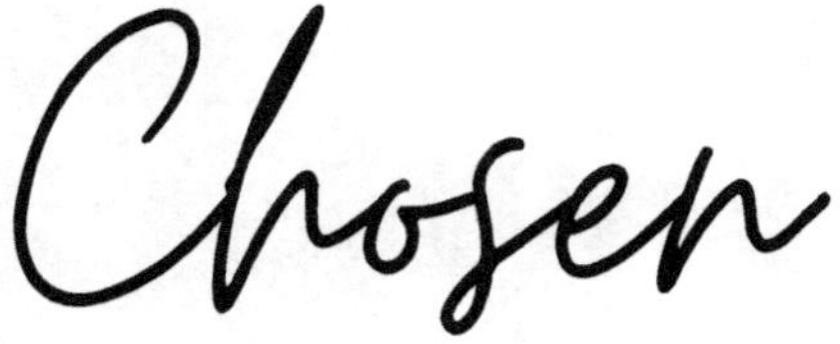

birth + faith through a doula lens

Katherine Leigh

Table of Contents

*For the moms needing truth to hold on to as
a lens for this season,*

*For the birth workers needing hope to rely
on as a stronghold for this holy work in the
space between the womb and the world,*

*With thanks to my two boys, who have
shown me such grace and joy in
motherhood; from whom I learn so much
about birth and life,*

*With gratitude for my Savior, Jesus Christ,
who was born to us in order to redeem us,*

*These words barely scratch the surface of
how interwoven our personal experiences of
birth and our understanding of theology,
the study of God, truly are.*

*Yet here they are, words wrapped in book
form, as a gift, just for you.*

01 What Does It Mean To Be Chosen?

I gave birth facing backward and squatting in the passenger seat of our car, while parked in a grocery store parking lot. I felt invincible, empowered, like nothing could stop me. And although the situation and timing en route wasn't ideal, I was as prepared as I could be for childbirth, as I studied birth and prepared my body throughout my pregnancy, for this sprint-like marathon.

I felt close to God, a sweet juxtaposition of the not-yet and here-now which occurs in a pivotal moment of transition: moving into new roles for myself, as a new mother of two, and for my newborn, earthside. [1, 2]

What happened surprised me, but my unexpected car birth didn't surprise God. Before each of us takes our breath, or wakes up each day, God goes before us and knows our steps. He chose us for the tasks before us. This includes childbirth. He knows the details of your pain, your labor, your baby- all of it. He is there, in the labor room (or car!).

Birth is a powerful, transformational moment in a mother's life, and it does us good to learn of it. No matter whether you are to give birth in nine months, maybe will someday, or had ten or more years ago, no matter where and with whom you choose to give birth, be it at a hospital, at a birth center, at home, or with a midwife or doctor or nobody else at all;

The concept of birth in the biblical narrative is a powerful illustration which can transform your view of God and shed light on how He dwells within and around us, how He chooses us, and how this changes the way we view childbirth.

We are chosen for the season of childbearing. And by our willingness, or perhaps despite our anxiety about the discomforts that can come in pregnancy, God creates new life within us - we become conduits for His creation. As Christian women - birth workers and mothers alike - to learn more about God, we must learn more about what He creates, and we must understand our role as conduits, vessels for His creation of a new life. This includes the process of labor and childbirth.

We learn more of birth; we learn more of God [3]. For He created us in His image, and in order to step fully into the role He planned for us we create, also. We are hardwired to create and reflect His image. So we learn about His design of the process of birth, and we learn about our role as His chosen work of art in His greater story, the facet in which a child is born into a family. Into His family. We are conduits for His creation, and in childbirth, we step into the greater biblical narrative. As He creates new life, we reflect on how the process mirrors our own experiences in pregnancy.

Have you ever thought of that, creating being similar to pregnancy? [4] The morning sickness and saltine crackers, the heavy days, the living being inside you, all as conduits for creation? [5] God created the land and the seas, and we humble ourselves in pregnancy and become the vessels for new life within. We trade everyday comfort for sickness and pain in an effort to be the vehicle for more of God's glory and grace in the world --- We are the created vessel, the conduit, for God's design. A new life made in His image.

God created us. And He invites us into the creation process by giving us the gift of pregnancy, by choosing us to be vessels for His creation, His masterpiece: new life in the womb. We humbly (and sometimes in agony) accept. The juxtaposition between not-yet and here-now that occurs in childbirth, the sweet transitional moment when your baby crowns and the heavens groan in glory --- He walks beside you, and He walks before you and meets you there.

You are *chosen* by the Most High, mama.

Moreover, if your birth was tragic, unexpected, or covered in loss, know that grief and thanks can coexist [6]; grace meets you here. (We will talk more about this in chapter 6).

Childbirth is theological [7]; God chose you for the season, and you do well by learning more about God and what He says about birth in order to fully step into your role. Birth isn't something that is done to you or just happens to you. It is an invitation from the Almighty to become conduits for His creation.

Yes, we mothers are in fact chosen for the season of childbearing, and God uses this season to bend our hearts toward Him as He creates new life within us.

Let us continue to redeem the fear-based cultural knowledge of labor and birth and replace it with purpose and truth through what God reveals to us in His word.

Let us celebrate our part and purpose in childbirth, no matter the type of birth had, and for every outcome.

Whether you plan to have a natural, medicated, or cesarean birth, you give birth to new life that God knit in your womb, and this is a beautiful part of God's design for us.

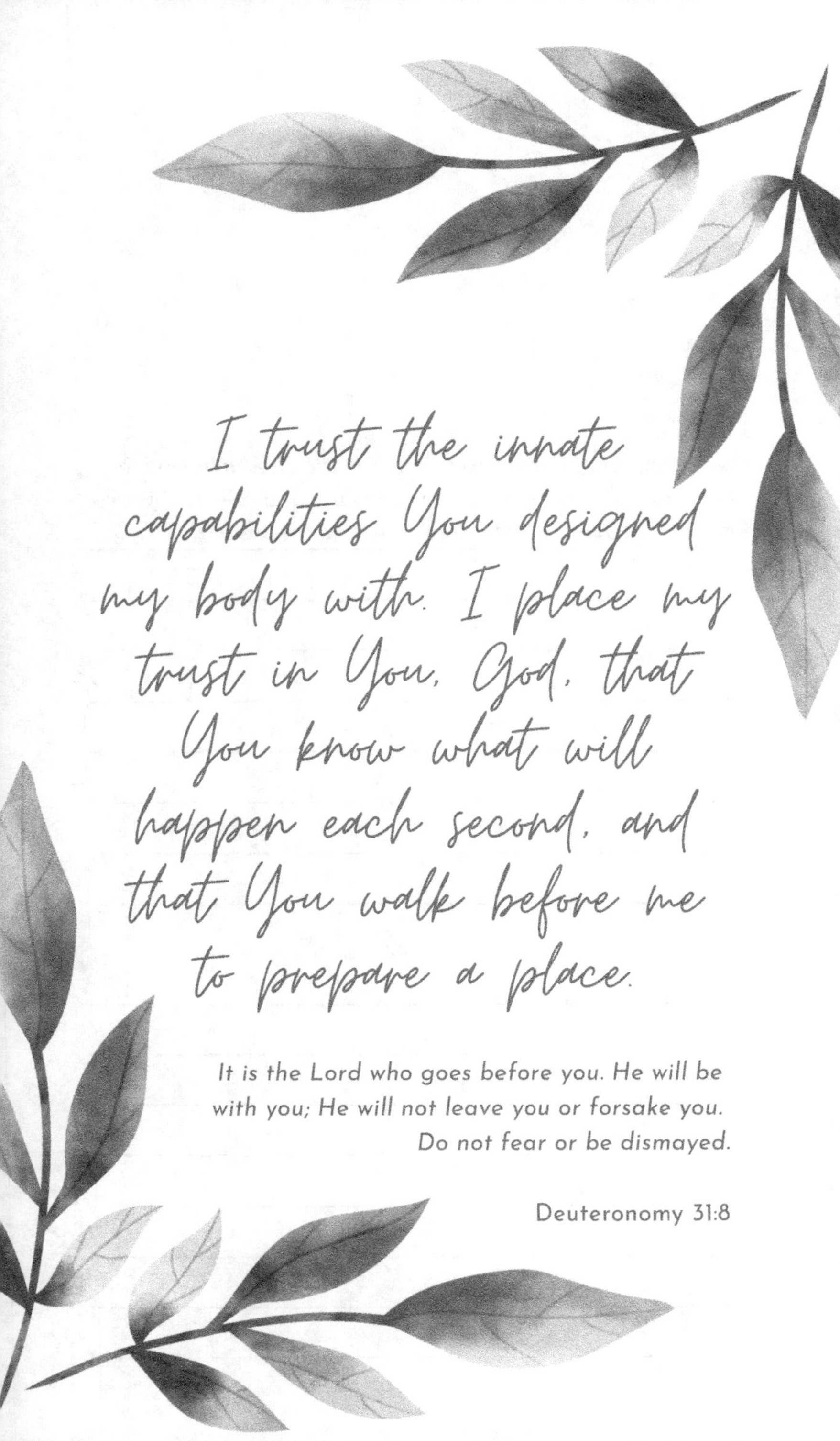

I trust the innate capabilities You designed my body with. I place my trust in You, God, that You know what will happen each second, and that You walk before me to prepare a place.

It is the Lord who goes before you. He will be with you; He will not leave you or forsake you. Do not fear or be dismayed.

Deuteronomy 31:8

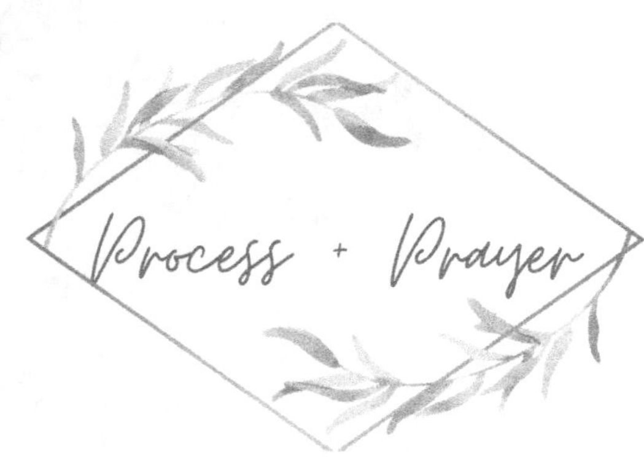

Take a few minutes to reflect on how being Chosen by God for this season affects how you move forward, and celebrate your pregnancy. Write a prayer to God for this gift.

02 Transform Your Pregnancy

Pregnancy can be so difficult, and we can so easily forget just how amazing pregnancy is. How amazing it is to know that you are chosen by God for this precious season, as well as how that transforms the way you think of and walk through your pregnancy in faith. If you're feeling sick, discouraged, or down about the physical or emotional symptoms that so often come along with pregnancy, let me help encourage you, by sharing how being chosen transforms your pregnancy. [1]

What a marvelous thought it is when we allow ourselves to dwell on it---that God entrusted a little person's life to you, that He is molding a child made in His image in your womb [2]. A new life. Let's rest in this thought for a few minutes, of what an incredible gift and honor this is, to be invited into God's design for new life... It is grace, and it is a miracle...

We are invited into the process of God's creation, and in it, we become the vessel for His miracle. Pregnancy is that life-giving vessel, a nine-month journey into a new reality for your family.

Seeing your pregnancy in the light of the gospel absolutely changes the way you view it. Because the little miracle, the new life in your womb, was chosen by God for your family at this exact time.

And you, mama, were chosen by God to enter into the process of housing---of becoming a vessel---of one of His miracles, a precious child.

The child whose heart beats at just 21 days from fertilization, before you can even confirm a positive pregnancy test [3].

The child, whom is the reason for your morning sickness and crackers in your purse, the new life your body is currently sustaining by God's grace, is such a beautiful gift. New life is redemptive, and new life is grace.

Let's explore more about how Scripture transforms your pregnancy; We all know that God values life, and the psalmist confirms this and declares in Psalm 139:13: "For You formed my inward parts; you knitted me together in my mother's womb (ESV)."

It is in the secret place, inside a mother's womb, that new life is created. There is also confirmation of this throughout the Bible.

Consider Luke 1. When Mary found out she was pregnant with Jesus, the coming Savior, she left for her cousin Elizabeth's home for a number of months.

Upon her arrival, something spectacular happened that brings pregnancy into a gospel light:"And when Elizabeth heard the greeting of Mary, the baby leaped in her womb. And Elizabeth was filled with the Holy Spirit" (Luke 1:41)

This baby grew up to be John the Baptist, Jesus's older cousin who paved the way for the Lord and baptized Jesus at the beginning of His earthly ministry (Matthew 3:13-17).

Knowing you are chosen, just as Mary and Elizabeth were, transforms how you view your pregnancy. God values pregnancy, as He values His children from the moment of conception to their last breath on this side of eternity [4].

More frequent bathroom breaks due to our ever-increasing bellies seen no longer as interruptions to our everyday but as welcome minutes of respite, reminders to take a breath and pray for our children growing and what God is doing in our lives.

The onset of labor is seen as a gift and invitation into God's creative process, a pivotal moment in one's life, rather than a fearful emergency –because in all this, we know Jesus walks with us.

Yes, throughout pregnancy, and yes, even in labor. By His presence, we have no reason to fear. By the grace of Jesus Christ, our pregnancy is redeemed as celebration.

We are walking through our days leading to motherhood no longer in fear, but in daily communion with and prayer to Jesus Christ, knowing that He will carry us through the pivotal events to come.

The gospel redeems and transforms pregnancy, and our lives are proof of this.

You are *chosen* for this season, mama. Know this well.

In light of the cross, the fear of pregnancy is replaced with truth of what Jesus is doing in us and through us – as vessels for His creation. He transforms our lives with salvation [4].

If or when He blesses us with childbearing, *He will transform us through it.* He is faithful.

And for those of us who have experienced loss, I will speak

to this in chapter 6 - please do not be discouraged!

Jesus knew this well, as He is at once human and fully God come to earth; His life and ministry outlined in the Gospels shows how He values us.

If we continue to look at pregnancy through a gospel lens, we learn that there is great joy to be had in the process, notably in us being invited into God's process of creation as vessels for His glory to be made known.

The gospel takes the uncomfortable moments of pregnancy and redeems the picture for us.

The gospel turns the picture of pregnancy into one of promise, of new life.

The gospel redeems pregnancy [5]; it is no longer nine months of our lives to fear or to be stuck in discontent in how our bodies our changing (*for better or worse – considering stretch marks!*)

In light of the redemption of the cross, we can exchange our sometimes negative views of pregnancy for ones of grace [5].

Because of the cross, the discomfort of a growing belly is now seen as the grace of a fruitful womb.

Morning sickness woes are seen as glory that pregnancy is progressing as God designed and our bodies are housing new life.

Stretch marks are transformed into battle wounds,

evidence of the beauty in the design of our bodies, capable of carrying life; displayed long after our children are born.

Pregnancy in light of the gospel is an honor and a gift, and Jesus celebrates every new life with us – from conception to birth and beyond.

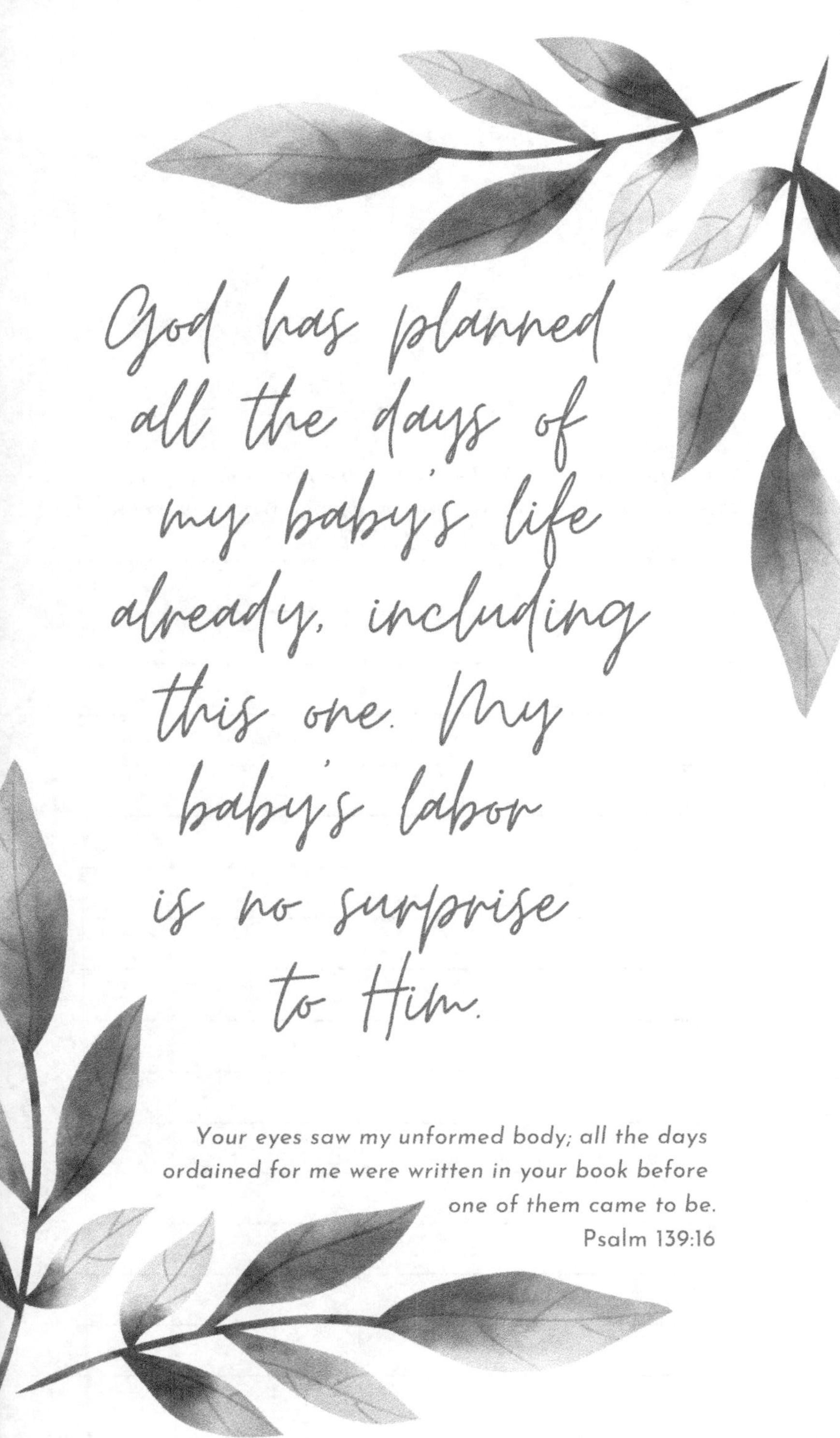

God has planned all the days of my baby's life already, including this one. My baby's labor is no surprise to Him.

Your eyes saw my unformed body; all the days ordained for me were written in your book before one of them came to be.
Psalm 139:16

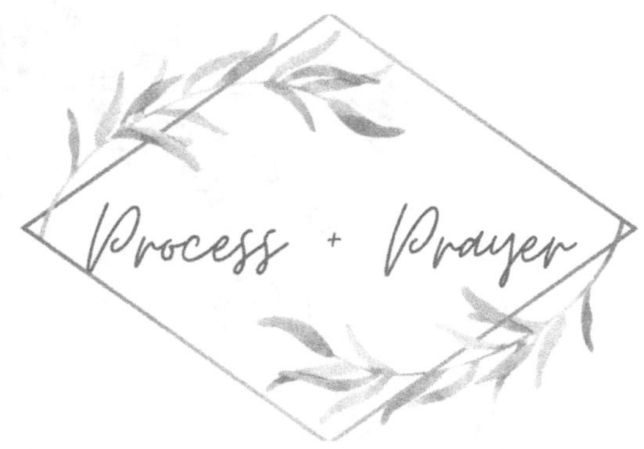

Take a few minutes to reflect on how being chosen by God for this season affects your views of pregnancy. Write a prayer to God for this gift.

____

____

____

____

____

____

____

____

____

____

____

____

____

____

____

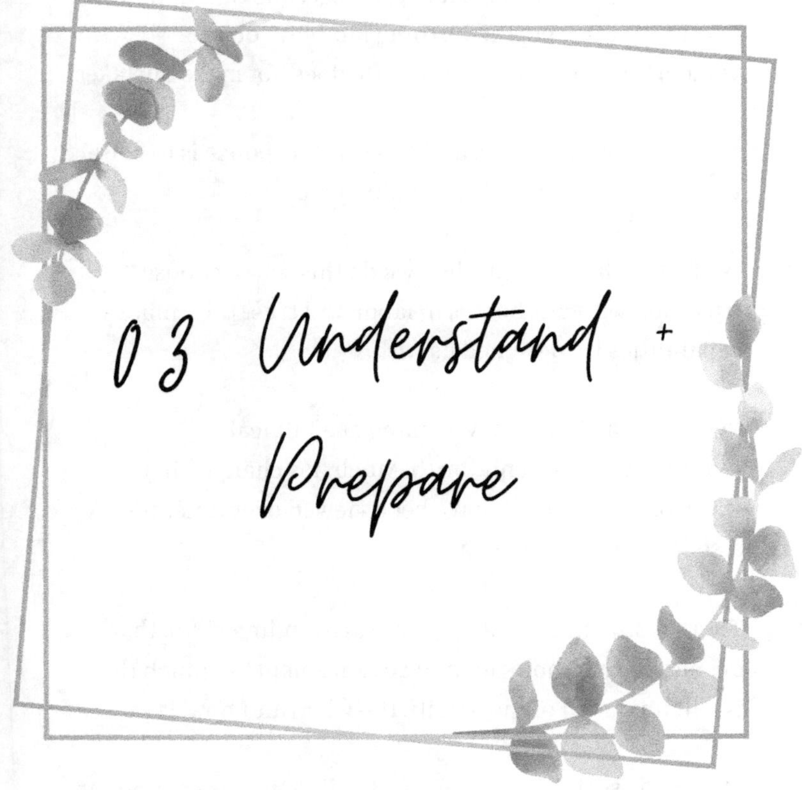
03 Understand +
Prepare

Can you see now how you are chosen by God for this precious season, that of bringing new life into the world?

While it's obvious that women were created biologically to bear children to carry on His creation, it can be easy to forget.

Easy to forget this incredible privilege, one that honors God and empowers the birthing mother. You are wonderfully made by God, and He does not make mistakes.

You are chosen by Him, and a natural response is to better understand this task He set before you.

We further honor God when we do this, as we choose to trust God with our bodies in labor and trust the innate capabilities He designed us with.

Yet it can easily get hazy, looking at a biblical understanding for childbirth. Much has changed in the way women and birth have been viewed over time, and we also have so much to learn.

There is still an aura of mystery surrounding birth, that despite the technologies and advancements so much that is still unknown of the details, the when and how. [1]

Mystery is sustained, as well as the discomforts common in pregnancy and labor. What we cannot control is further put into a box in an attempt to rein in the process, a man-made antidote to fear about God's design. And in this we limit ourselves.

So we learn and we study. And knowing that we are chosen

by God for this season means that we must also understand the process of birth He created. For there is power in knowledge, and there is impeccable strength in God's design. This prompts us to better prepare for this season of pregnancy and birth.

To put it in a greater biblical light, we can see childbirth as God's mercy for us [2]. For in Genesis, we read that God chose to give Adam and Eve the gift to multiply, even after they sinned against Him, although they deserved death.

God chose life in the garden, and He continues to choose life for us today---as He invites us directly into the birth process, in how He created and designed women.

As Gloria Furman wrote once for the Gospel Coalition, *life is a precious gift from a holy and just God.* [3, empahsis mine]

And as you continue to celebrate your part in birth, you naturally continue to learn about birth: the physiological process, the stages and progression of labor, the common discomforts in pregnancy, or different support persons, positions or biblical affirmations or even distractions to aide you in your labor.

Knowing your part in birth prompts you to better understand and prepare for labor and childbirth itself. Knowing that God chose you for this season shifts your view on childbirth from one of fear to one of faith, from one of anxiety to one of peace, from one of anger to one of joy. *It is truly possible!*

By learning about birth to prepare yourself alongside

learning that you are chosen for this season, you are celebrating your role and purpose in birth by seeking what God says about women, about childbirth, and most importantly, about Himself.

The noise in our world today surrounding a fear-based culture of childbirth can be silenced by the overwhelming peace and knowledge that Christ bestows on us, as He chose us for this season.

It is too easy to fall into the trap of worldly thinking, that birth is something to suffer through. *Rather, it is something to marvel at.*

In fact, Scripture often relates birth to God and His chosen nation, Israel [4]. Yes, the nation of Israel, which He chose in order to further His kingdom on earth. And He continues to choose us, by the grace of Christ.

By learning of this greater arc in Scripture [5], that of the metaphor of birth and how God truly seeks His people, we only enhance our own peace of the process He designed. And we are prompted to continue to seek His wisdom in preparing for birth.

By learning of the physiology of birth, the stages of labor, the ways our bodies and each stage and minute of labor are purposefully designed by our very detailed creator God, we continue to marvel in faith, rather than tremble with fear.

Isn't that what we all want, at our core?

Not just to grit our teeth and get through it but to ease our fears and anxieties, to seek God and keep Him center in labor, as a child fresh from Him crowns earthside. Birth is a miracle and mystery all at once, and in this we . are invited into God's greater narrative.

In this we understand we are chosen and further seek His wisdom of how He designed our bodies and the birth process itself.

An expectant mother armed with knowledge and faith gains a powerful antidote to fear.

A birth worker who seeks to learn about her profession in a biblical light gives a gift to each mom she supports: That of walking alongside as a professional and a friend in faith, and meeting the mom's needs in this precious time.

There is truly a special bond gained by mothers in birth and the women who come alongside them to support.

Each birth is a moment like no other in history, as birth is unique each time a mother encounters it; gathering many factors and nuances while following a general, well-studied pattern,:that between not-yet and here-now, progressing in the stages of labor, each moment closer to meeting her child, her gift.

Being chosen prompts us to better understand and prepare for childbirth.

Whether it's by reading birth stories, learning the physiological process a woman's body undergoes in birth, hiring a doula and selecting your support persons, or asking all the questions when seeing your provider...

The more we learn, the more our faith sparks and the more prepared we are for this truly life-changing season.

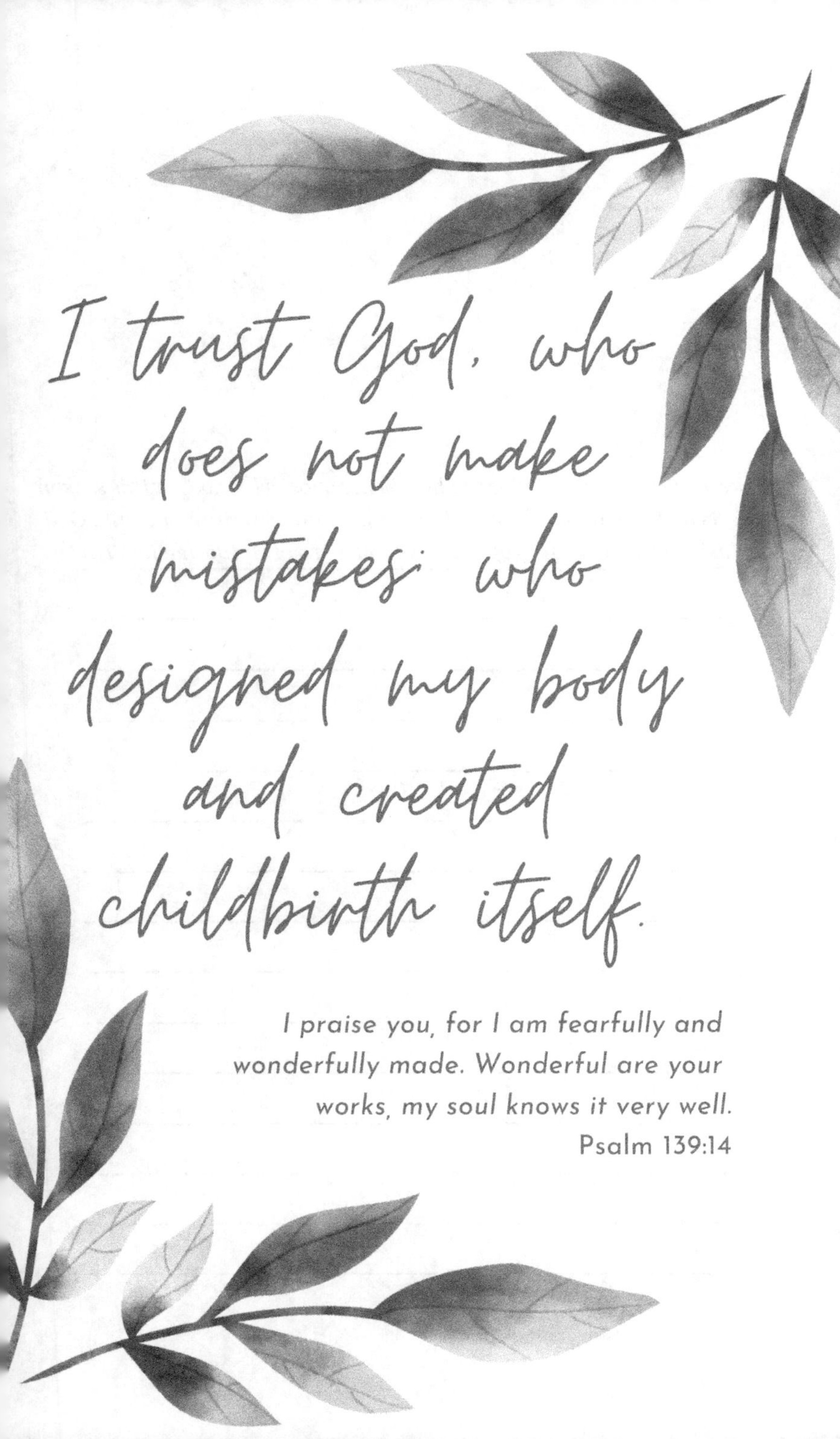

I trust God, who does not make mistakes; who designed my body and created childbirth itself.

I praise you, for I am fearfully and wonderfully made. Wonderful are your works, my soul knows it very well.
Psalm 139:14

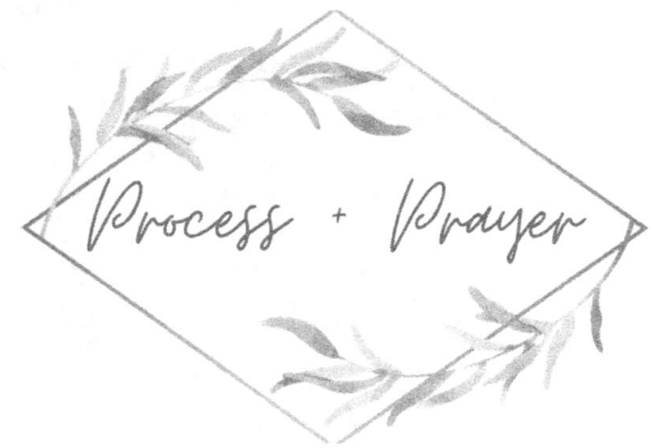

Take a few minutes to reflect on how being chosen by God for this season affects how you understand and prepare for birth. Write a prayer to God, asking Him to spark your faith as you learn of His design in birth.

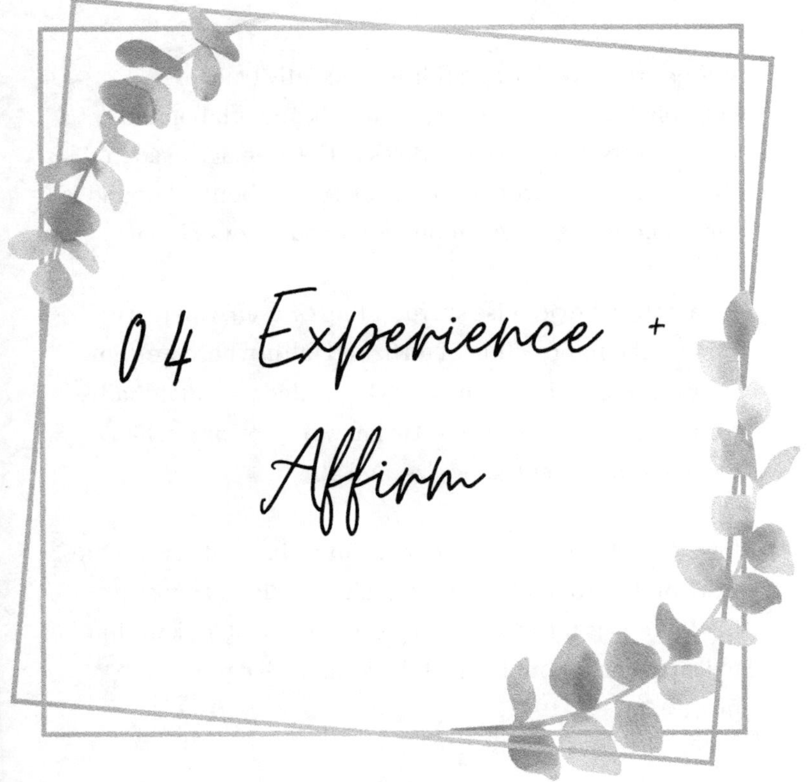

04 Experience + Affirm

While we can certainly learn of the childbirth process and prepare in a variety of ways, we also need to know how to apply this knowledge while in the throes of labor. It can be easy to get lost in the moment, yet be encouraged to dig deeper into your language and use of words. Namely, Biblical affirmations, which can greatly aid a mother's mind and spirit in the midst of labor. There's more to this than you may realize...

Words are powerful, and this is especially true for childbirth.The verbiage we use to talk about labor and birth affects how a woman views it; the verbiage used in the Scriptures in which God speaks to us about labor and birth, should have even more pull in our view of labor.

Remember the premise surrounding *Chosen*, where we explore the intersection of birth and faith, where we know in every fiber of our being that God called us individually, from our mothers womb --- He knew us---by name, hair color, temperament, shoe size, and all.

If God went to such great lengths for us in creation and the work of the cross, who designed birth itself and chose us to be His vessels for new life, why should we not look to Him to learn more about birth and take an active role in the process?

Further, as Christian mothers and birth workers, we have the privilege of being the vessels or support of a new life in this world... Why should we cheapen the experience by not planning for birth itself, the process that God designed?

In chapter 3, we learned about birth. And in this chapter, we affirm the process.

Know this: planning to have biblical affirmations on hand, as well as coping techniques and specialized support, such as your midwife, doula, or partner, is key.

For myself, as a Christian mom, I knew I wanted to honor my faith during labor. And in order to have a positive birth experience, I knew that affirmations were needed. Praying Scripture and keeping affirmation cards and phrases handy were perfect ways to have that positive experience.

Yes, birth affirmations are incredible tools for women to use in labor, and it's vital as a Christian woman that you find a faith source, if you choose to use them.

Because, in this fallen world we live in, there is a lot of verbiage surrounding birth is New Age and other-worldly; that is the noise we must instead filter to find God's truth.

To touch on some of the verbiage, we do not "trust birth itself" or see our bodies as a means to an end; rather, we place our trust in God.

For the Lord is our refuge and our strength. Not any method, plan, experience, training, or facility.

Read these next few affirmations: Do you hear the verbiage of inherent trust in ourselves and our bodies? Then pay attention to how I transformed them through a biblical lens.

Now we have a script to remember in the throes of labor, which points us to Christ:

For my body is capable and strong...*by God's design.*

I can do this....*by the grace of Christ.*

Fear has no place...*because perfect love cast it out.*

Even though I feel overwhelmed and mentally drained....*Christ gives me strength to keep on.*

I am in pain....*but God has a purpose.*

Even Isaiah 66:9 states, "I will not cause pain without allowing something new to be born."

So we honor Him in our birth by affirming that we are chosen for this moment, for this child, for this labor. In fact, knowing we are chosen completely transforms the way we experience and affirm labor, the process that God designed.

Remember chapters 2 and 3:

Because of Christ, we can have peace in the process, in place of anxiety.

Because of Christ, we can feel awe in the process, in place of fear.

Because of Christ, pain is seen as glory [1] and grace in that our bodies are working as God designed.

And ultimately, in this a new life enters the world.

We use and repeat simple, biblical affirmations while in the throes of labor; by doing so, we also keep our mind, soul, and spirit, in check with the Holy Spirit.

We boast in Christ alone, not in the type of birth we have. For He deserves all the praise.

Because while childbirth is unique for each woman and child, understanding the general process and finding ways to walk through the time positively – no matter the type of birth you are having – is proven to ease fears and anxieties of the unknown.

Having some key phrases and scriptures memorized is proven to be instrumental as an aide in labor [2]; prayer and the communion with God it brings usher a peace into the moment that wasn't possible prior.

Because you are chosen by God for this season, you can experience and affirm labor and birth, the process He designed, in a way that honors Him.

By having biblical affirmations on hand or memorized, you can swiftly bring Christ into the labor room and focus on the strength He gives you each moment, each contraction, each breath.

As a doula or birth worker, giving a mama the option of having affirmation cards for labor and creating those together if she chooses is such a gift.

As a mother myself, I recall how important it was to be mindful and present in the throes of my surprising car labor (*remember the story in chapter 1!*).

It's the reason each chapter ends with a biblical affirmation - to stress the importance of the ways we prepare, which trickle into and paint our experiences, especially as Christian women.

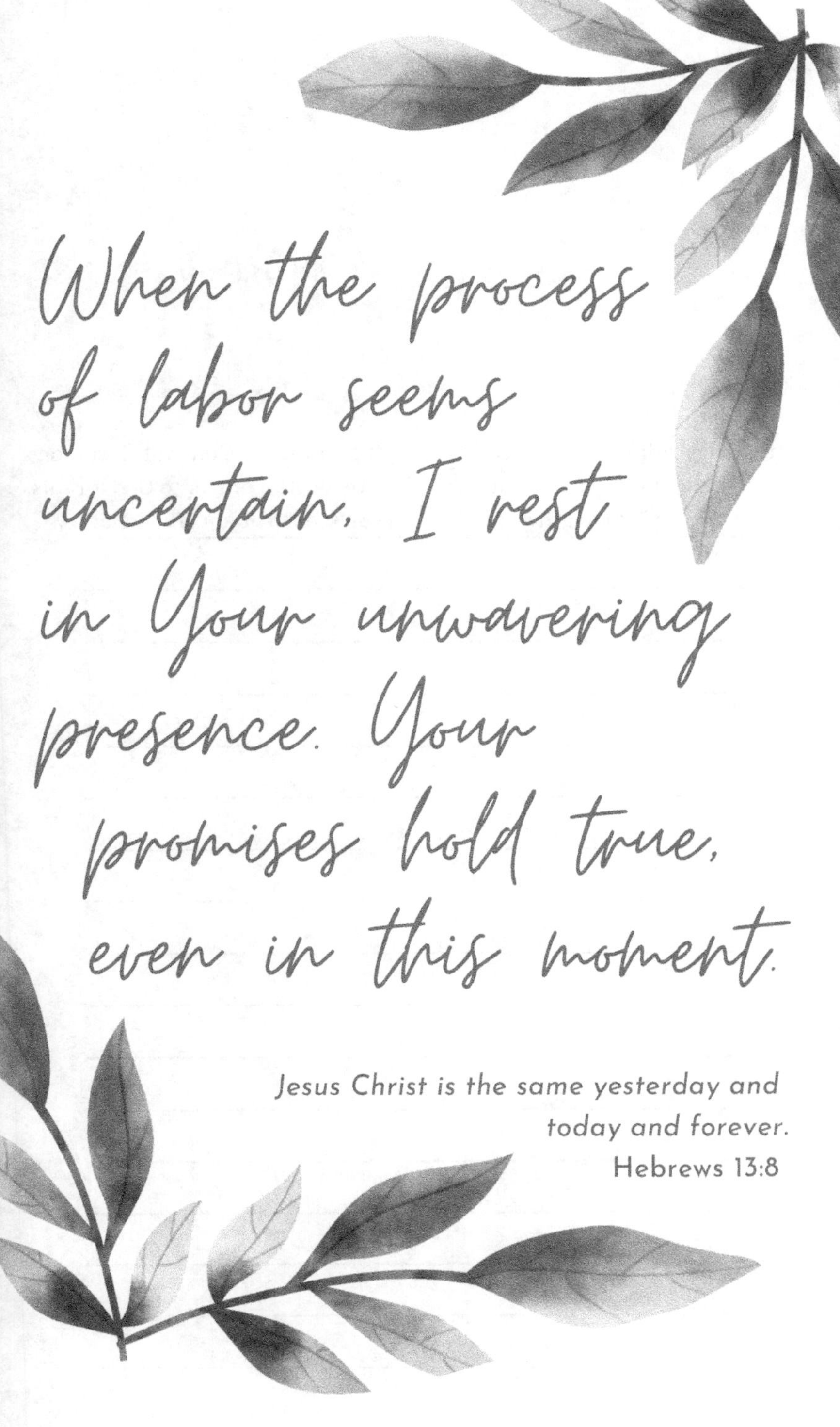

When the process of labor seems uncertain, I rest in Your unwavering presence. Your promises hold true, even in this moment.

Jesus Christ is the same yesterday and today and forever.
Hebrews 13:8

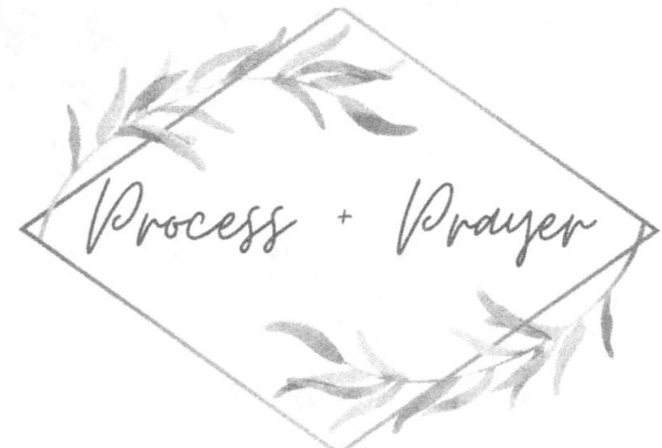

Take a few minutes to reflect on how being chosen by God for this season affects how you experience and affirm birth. Write a prayer to God for this gift, asking Him to grow your faith as you seek to honor Him in labor.

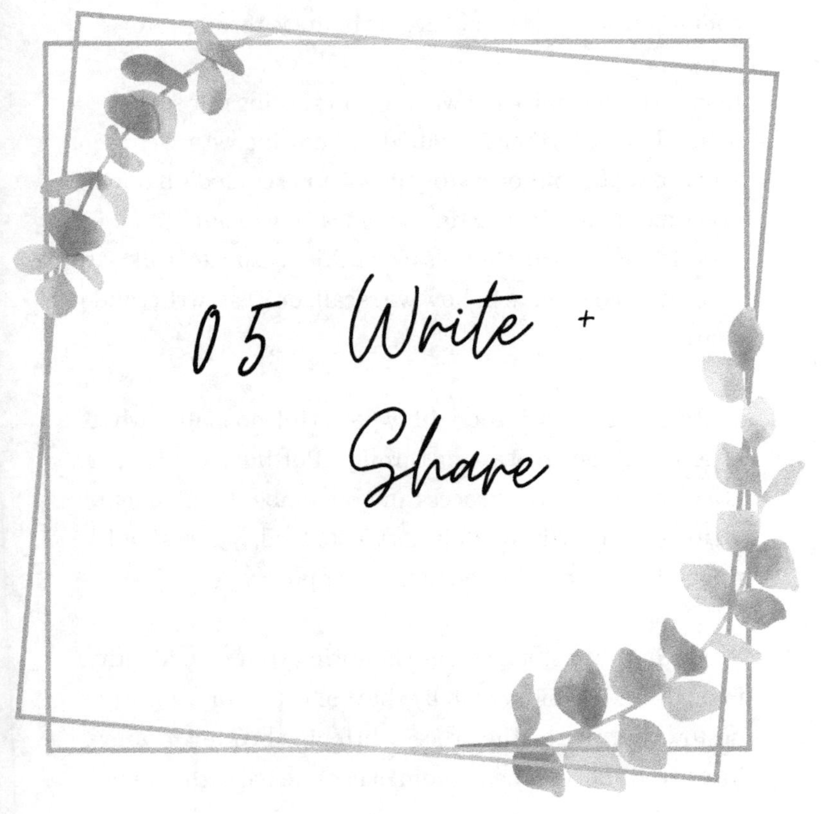

05 Write + Share

Childbirth is a moment in a woman's life that is unique every time she walks through it. It is very personal, very demanding, and a pivotal experience she will remember for the rest of her life.

One great way to record important moments in one's life is to journal and document them. And the greatest way we communicate and journal events in life is through story.

In fact, the act and art of writing and sharing our stories with others is further cemented by knowing we are chosen. You can write your own story down and see God's hand in every moment. Because He gives meaning to our experiences and He chooses us for this season, to walk with Him, to be coauthors in how we recall, process, write, and share.

Writing your story is incredibly powerful, no matter what experience you are walking through. Putting pen to paper is a way to honor the process and remember the moment. Writing your birth story allows you to heal, process, and remember your child's birth in an empowering way.

By writing your story, you are honoring your own identity in birth, and memory of it. By sharing your story, you are bestowing grace on the process, bringing healing to your heart, and sharing the wisdom of experience with others.

In *Walking on Water*, beloved author Madeleine L'Engle shares that "there is something healthily affirming about such structure, a promise that we have a part in the making of meaning. This is not a false promise or an unreal self control, but a promise that we are co-authors with God in the writing of our own story." [1]

Because ultimately, story is how God connects with us ----
the story of the promise and the blessing, seen in the
covenant with Israel and the covenant bestowed by grace
in Christ; the greater story of God's chosen people and how
we can see Him work in history and today. The story of
how God chooses us for this season and purpose.

You are chosen for your child, for your birth story, for this
moment. And knowing we are chosen prompts us to write
and share our stories of birth.

Story is how we relate to one another as human beings,
story is a part of our everyday mundane, and story is how
we remember and live. Stories are powerful and can
invoke tears, laughter, frustration, and so much more.
Stories are recognizable patterns, and it's in these patterns
that we find meaning. Story helps to make sense of life and
the world, to understand one's struggles or joys.

*Life is a story, and your child's life begins with a story, a
story of a birth.*

Even more, we are all wired for story . In her book *Rising
Strong*, Brene Brown emphasizes this in explaining how
when we hear a story from beginning to end, each line or
climax or plot twist, our brains release cortisol and
oxytocin [2] --- yes, oxytocin, the very same hormone
released by our pituitary glands during birth, the hormone
that causes contractions and stimulates a mother's milk
production.

*How incredibly beautiful and intricate and purposeful is
that?!* God designed our inner wirings to release the same
hormones while hearing a story that we also release in

childbirth and while nursing our fresh babe.

There is absolutely no mistake in this, mama. God designed the process, He chose you for this role, and He writes you into the greater story of His family by making you His daughter, and further, as you bear a child made in His image in the world.

We honor God, who chose us for this time, who designed our bodies so intricately, when we share how He has worked in our days, when we share our stories --- of birth, of life.

And it's at this moment, when we write or hear or share a story, that we can further connect, empathize, sympathize, and make meaning. *Story is literally in our DNA* [3].

Poet and Arielle Estoria shared at the 2019 hope*writers conference, a statement and a question: "*You are needed because your story is needed. There is always room for more because what is life anyway, except a collection of beautiful stories, a collection of your beautiful stories?*"[3]

Further, here are three simple reasons which illustrate importance of writing and sharing your story in community with others [4]:

To Process: Writing is truly therapeutic. By writing something down, you are more likely to remember it. And you are naming it. Giving experiences names is very powerful.

Writing your birth story causes you to think about what happened, and in this, you process what happened.

For Purpose: Writing is something that gives richer meaning to what we are walking through. In the context of childbirth, story helps to illustrate that experiences have a purpose: to enrich your life, or to learn from them. By writing out your birth story when it is still fresh in your mind, it helps you to remember why, what, how, when, and more.

To Remember: Memory can be a tricky thing in motherhood, as well as in heightened experiences, especially childbirth.

Ever heard of mom brain or pregnancy brain?

Writing things down helps you to remember --- it's simple yet painfully true. By writing a story as soon as possible after it happens, you will remember it better. The details, the feelings, the mundane or trauma of what happened.

Start your child's life by writing down his or her birth story. One day she or he may appreciate reading it and knowing the details;

And surely, mama, you will too.

Then share it!

Sharing your story is incredibly powerful. Sharing your birth story helps other mothers to know they are not alone. Sharing helps to validate your own experiences. Sharing your birth story can have a ripple effect much further than you'd ever dream.

Because stories travel and help us to know that we all

experience the same aches and joys to some degree or another [5].

Remember, we are wired for story, and it's how we make meaning in life.

We live best when we live in community; sharing stories is a natural outpouring of this [6].

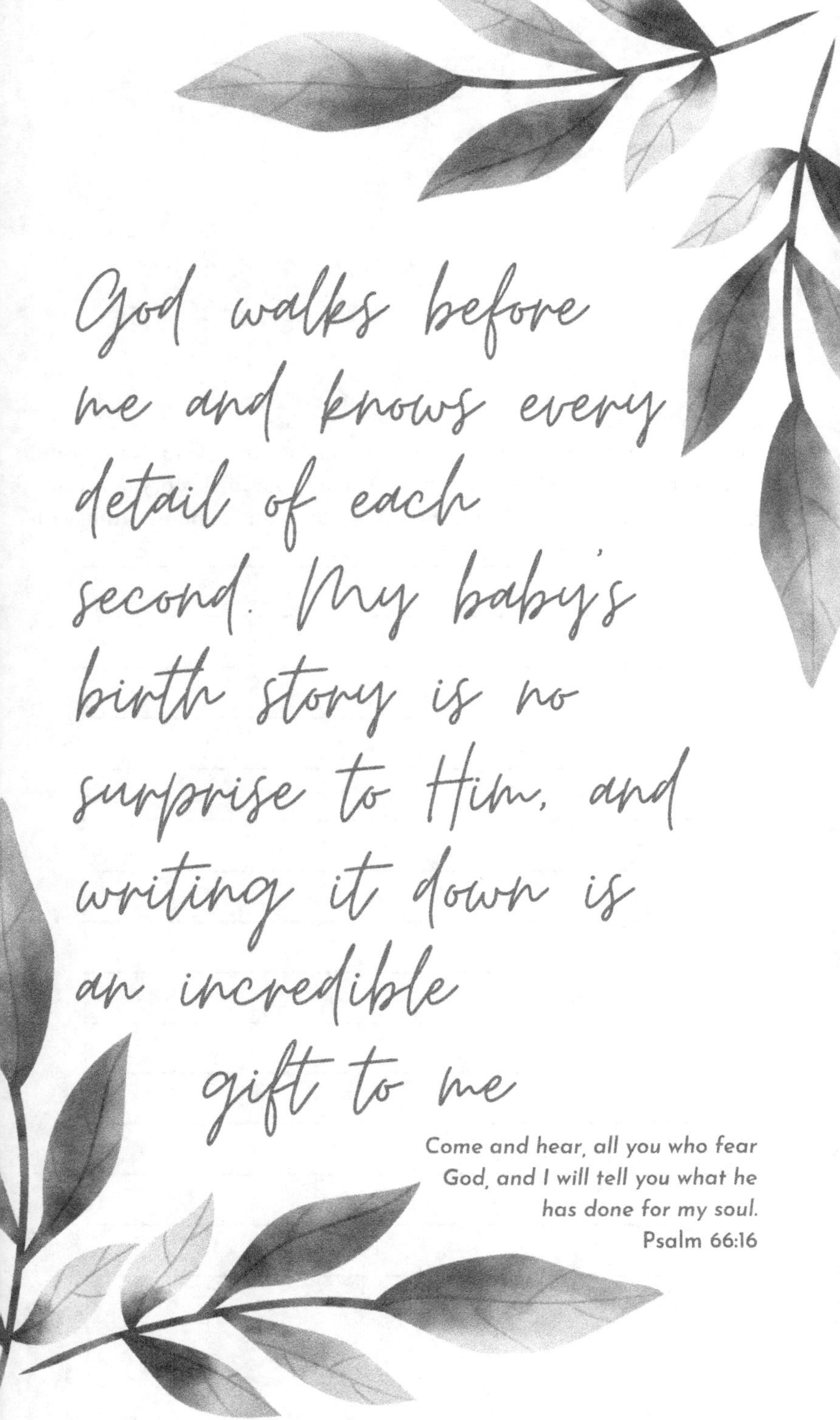
God walks before me and knows every detail of each second. My baby's birth story is no surprise to Him, and writing it down is an incredible gift to me

Come and hear, all you who fear God, and I will tell you what he has done for my soul.
Psalm 66:16

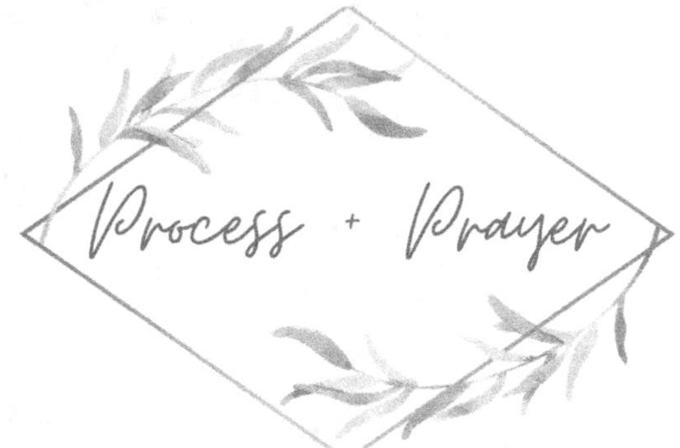

Take a few minutes to reflect on how being chosen by God for this season affects how you recall, process, write + share your birth story. Write a prayer to God, thanking Him for the gift of words, for communicating with us through His story of Scripture.

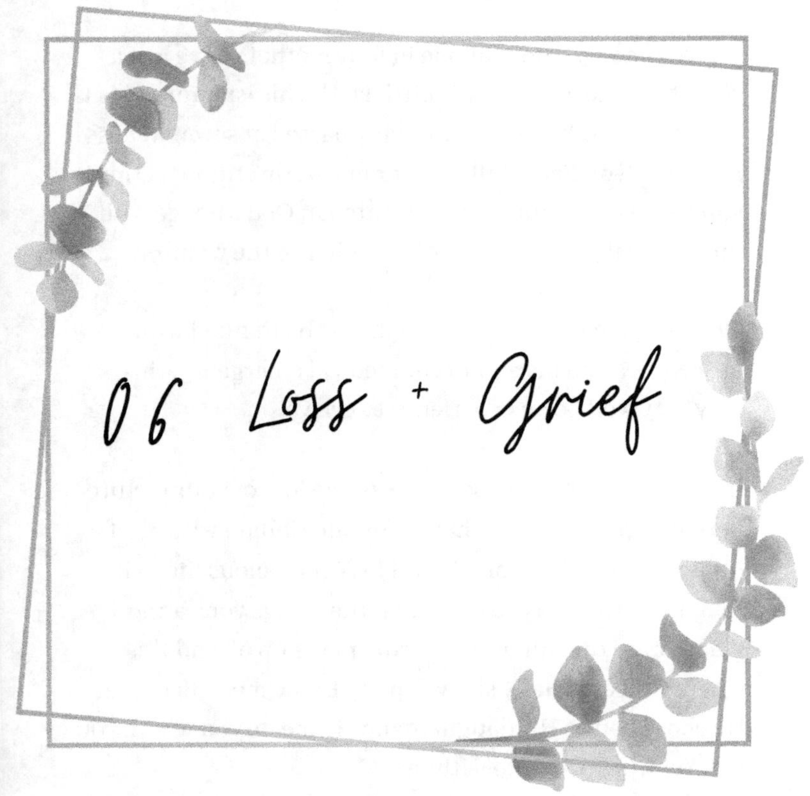

06 Loss + Grief

Grief is an undeniable part of the human experience and should never be stifled. There are healthy ways to grieve, and there are reasons it is necessary to allow ourselves to do so. This is a reality for many of the women surrounding us each day --- mothers, sisters, friends. *Do you know your neighbor well enough?*

It is commonly said that one in four mothers have lost a child to miscarriage or stillbirth [1,3]. This isn't rare; this is a daily reality. Whether your baby passed at seven weeks gestation, you had a full-term or mid-term stillbirth, this is still the loss of a human life, created in God's image with intrinsic value, which He knit together in the womb.

Or, if you experienced a traumatizing birth filled with obscenities and discomfort or medical emergency, this may very well be an experience to grieve.

In a traumatic birth experience, in the loss of your picture-perfect birth plan in exchange for one riddled with grief, unmet expectations, or a literal loss of precious life--- It's tough yet necessary to learn that the things you cannot plan for are the things life is truly made up of, and this is where God especially shows up [2]. In the mess. Because He chose you as His daughter and He meets you where you are. Yet what do we do with that?

Pressing in, a better question becomes this: *What do we do when we face the loss of our ideal birth, the loss of a human life, the loss of the hopes of what could be...even when we know that God chooses us?*

In short, we grieve. Yes, we grieve, even more so when we know that we are chosen by God as His daughter for this truth trickles into our response of everything we experience --- surely including grief.

The loss of a child should never be taboo, and knowing we are chosen affects this. Because although you haven't met that child on this side of heaven, that child is fully alive in Christ in heaven [4]. And God still chooses her. And He still chose you to be her mother.

Not having your child in your arms does not make you any less of a mother, and it doesn't make your child any less of a child made in God's image. Chosen.

Yet still, how do we walk forward in this reality, one of loss and grief?

Here are some tangible ways to acknowledge yourself or your friend in her loss and grief [5]:
- Celebrate life --- whether it was weeks of gestation, or minutes earthside.
- Say the child's name (and name her!).
- Affirm that she existed, mattered, is loved, and is full of life in heaven.
- And most of all, know that this is not our home and one day you will see her again.

Acknowledge your baby or your friends baby, and be willing to talk if invited to or when you are ready. Words heal.

And just because we grieve a loss doesn't mean we aren't also thankful that there is another name, another child, that belongs to us, whom we do know on this side of eternity.

With this point, this chapter could easily be titled "What Not To Say To A Woman Experiencing Miscarriage, Stillbirth, or a Traumatic Birth," because gratefulness for the child you have is often an excuse for ignoring the traumatic experience you are walking through (or so often I've been told). Also, please don't tell this to a grieving mother.

While it may be tempting to shove emotions away, this is a toxic train of thought. Luke 19:40 states, *"If they keep quiet, the stones will cry out (NIV)."*

If we remain silent and fail to grieve and give thanks to, or even at the very least we can muster, to acknowledge God in that juxtaposition this places us in, we also fail to see God at work in it. We bury the emotions and hurt ourselves further in the process, delaying our healing. We refuse to talk about reality, and again, we quietly bury our emotions. We fester, and we don't allow God in the door.

This is not a way to live.

This applies to much of the human experience --- especially to the loss of an ideal birth or the loss of a child --- especially to our experiences of grief.

God is in the grief of unmet expectations. Yet we are still to give thanks for His sovereignty. [2]

Because even so, you know that you are chosen by God as His precious child and to be His vessel for new life. And yes, mama, your child does have a full life in Christ in heaven, even when you aren't holding her in your arms earthside. It is a hard yet joyful reality and tension to live in. The not-yet, where you long to know your child while understanding that she has never known pain, loss, or grief, the way she would on this side of heaven...this spot of in-between is plain hard. There is no way around it.

The brokenness that comes from the unexpected --- when our plans go awry --- can be debilitating. Broken pieces can become muddled in the grief of real life. Yet God is in the midst, He is in the outcome, and He will walk you through the grieving process. He knows your situation before you live it, and He is with you. Allow the pain then release it to God as He mends your broken heart.

God mends reality and bestows grace. Indeed, grief and thanks can coexist.

Your grief does not overshadow God's unwavering promise. Your experience does not mean God has abandoned you.

Grieve the experience but give thanks for His sovereignty. You can be grateful for a healthy baby and also feel the loss of the birth you wanted. You can still see grace in the face of Jesus, in community, in love in action, in your neighbors becoming the hands and feet of Christ in a time you so desperately need them, as you grieve the passing of a child. In Christ, you can find a gentle guide, a shepherd who comes alongside you through all the pains of life. Including this pain.

If your birth plans went awry, know this: writing your story has power (as explored in chapter 5), counseling is a strength for your hard moments, and prayer is your anchor in the storm to keep you grounded in faith as you walk forward.

One final practice for you as you walk through grief: putting to pen the thoughts in your mind is eye-opening. I liken this to David lamenting in the Psalms; while being thankful for life and God's sovereignty, you honor where you are in the grief.

This does not make you weak, nor is it something to be ashamed of. This is hard, and help is OK. It's important to do this in order to more fully see God's fingerprints all over the birth we grieve, to remedy our view of faith and God's sovereignty over the unexpected in life. Because while childbirth itself is inevitable, what happens during it is ultimately unexpected; there is no way to know how it will unfold. Life doesn't go as planned.

Birth is unique to the mom and baby involved --- no two births are alike. As mothers of faith, we can accept this reality, and choose to grieve the unexpected birth outcome, rather than cling tightly to our plans gone awry, ultimately creating contempt in our hearts. The unexpected becomes the undeniable: a birth that didn't go as planned becomes the birth in which we see God's right hand keeping us safe, because He walks before us and prepares a way.

Birth, even when grief comes, is indeed a powerful experience and is a way for us to enter the narrative of Christ, the story of God's chosen people, which includes you and which includes this unexpected outcome you live in.

Grief and thanks can and do walk hand in hand.

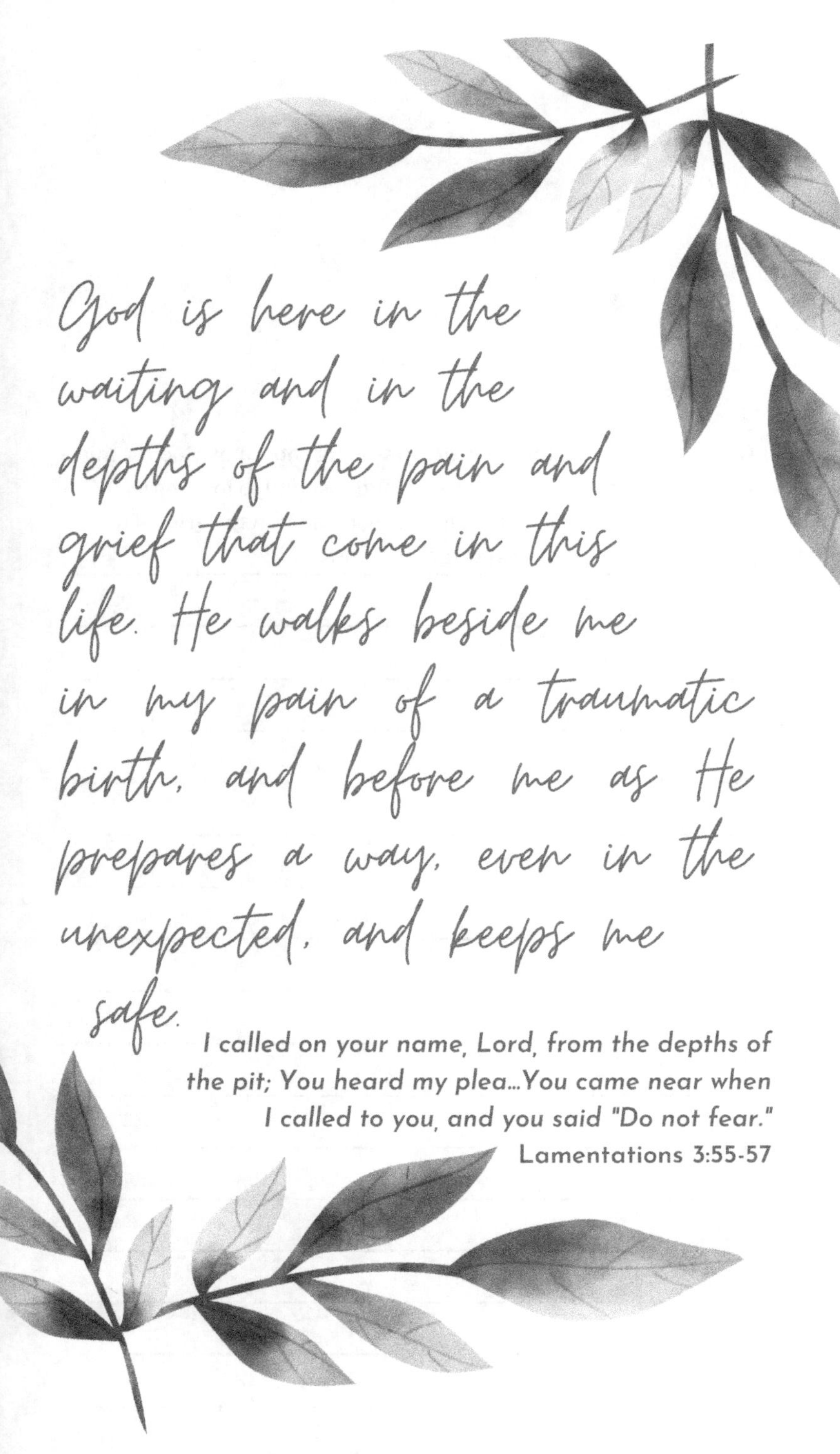
God is here in the waiting and in the depths of the pain and grief that come in this life. He walks beside me in my pain of a traumatic birth, and before me as He prepares a way, even in the unexpected, and keeps me safe.

I called on your name, Lord, from the depths of the pit; You heard my plea...You came near when I called to you, and you said "Do not fear."
Lamentations 3:55-57

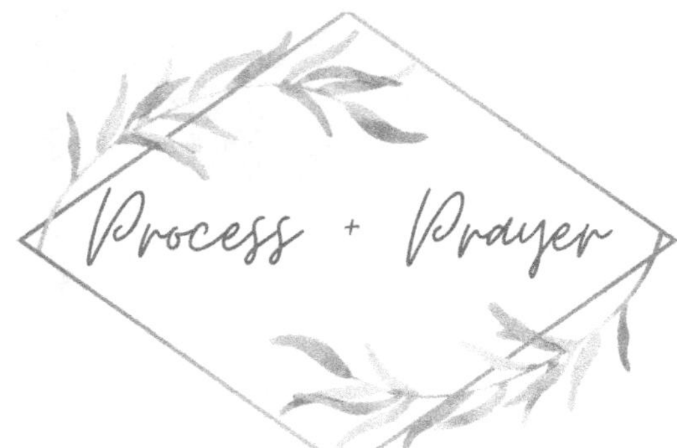

Take a few minutes to reflect on how being chosen by God for this season affects how you walk through and respond to loss + grief. Write a prayer to God, thanking Him for being present in the grief of unmet expectations + loss.

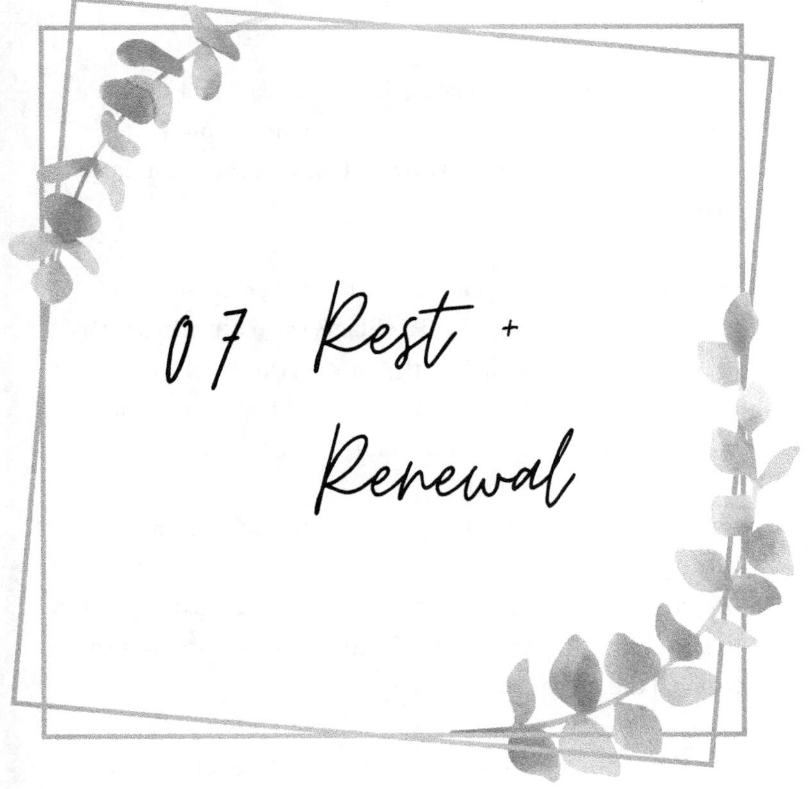

07 Rest + Renewal

With nowhere else to turn, I did the best I could at the time with what I had in front of me. I read all the books, had all the teas and cookies, memorized the details of the stages of labor and birth, stocked my freezer full of meals, ate all the recommended foods---the list of preparation goes on. But truly, nothing prepares anyone for this, for what happened to my mind and body, postpartum with my second earthside babe. [1]

There's much to tell, yet sometimes it doesn't feel so. Since my son was born in the car en route to the hospital, well, nobody knew what to do with us. (Read chapter 1 for parts of the story).

My first moments postpartum with a newborn, that time we are told so often we need a village, wasn't turning out as planned. With us being healthy, moving, and alert fairly immediately after birth, everything that happened around us felt unnecessary, like too much.

I just wanted to be able to take care of my baby in the best way I knew how and utilize all the research and preparation I had collected the past months. I just wanted to be at home as a family, nestle into my new normal, away from all the noise around me.

And there lies the issue: *the noise around me.* There was too much, and in it, my own voice felt muffled.

Yet when your voice feels muffled, the village seems lost. And what does a new mother do when that happens?

A village for postpartum mothers can never happen in a world where we muffle the voices of those crying out for , help, fail to follow-up often and continue to offer ourselves as help after babe is born.

Truly, community care is needed even more than self-care, especially in such a fragile, precious time as postpartum.

It takes a village, and as Christian women, we need to step up, come alongside new moms, and become the community we've always wanted, helping postpartum moms with needs and being that support, in whichever way fits her needs best.

If that postpartum mom is you, know that you do need that village for rest and renewal in this time. *And here's why.*

The postpartum period in a mother's life is a precious time that should be guarded with care. Knowing that we are chosen by God for this season drives this point even further; *we should honor Him in how we rest and heal in community.*

The postpartum period isn't just the first six weeks after a baby is born either --- commonly known as the fourth trimester. In fact, many sources argue that it extends through the first year, even the first three years, of a baby's life [2] --- because it takes time for our bodies to recover, no matter the type of birth.

Mama, you are chosen by God for this precious season of pregnancy, birth, and the days with a fresh babe, as well as those to come in motherhood. Steward this time well by learning about the importance of rest, the importance of community and your village, and the importance of caring for your whole mind, body, and spirit during this time.

Looking further to Scripture, in John 15:4-5 (NIV) Jesus sums up how best to care for yourself: "Abide in me, and I in you. As the branch cannot bear fruit by itself, unless it abides in the vine, neither can you, unless you abide in me. I am the vine; you are the branches. Whoever abides in me and I in him, he it is that bears much fruit, for apart from me you can do nothing."

We are to remain, be present, be held, and be kept continually by Jesus Christ in order to produce lives that glorify Him [3]. This can especially be done in the postpartum period, as this is a precious time in a woman's life that forces her to slow down to listen to her baby and her body as both recover from the rigors of childbirth.

By resting in Him and being fully present in our days, we align our desires and actions with His. spiritual fruit flourishes. Even if they are like whispers – Jesus hears you and meets you there. Every minute has a purpose!

As we sink into God, we can savor the life-giving relationships of those around us, and gain encouragement from others during postpartum. For we were created for community, as humans created in God's image; He designed us to spend time with and bear with one another, love one another, lift one another up, and come alongside to support one other the way we long to be cared for [4]. Rest in Christ, and seek help and support through your community. This community, or village, is vital for a well-rounded life in every circumstance --- it is by God's design!

It takes a village, and as moms with fresh babes, we need to realize that we can't do this alone; we need Jesus, we need prayer, and we, in fact, need a village.

"It takes a village" is traditionally an African proverb, illustrating that an entire community of people must interact with children for those children to grow and learn in a safe and healthy environment [5]. The village looks out for one another. The village is a community, a family, doing life together.

This can be translated into every facet of the human exprience. And as women of faith, this is what we are called to – encouraging one another, living in community. It is a necessary fact of being human – people need people in order to thrive.

The village, or community, a new postpartum mother needs is more than just a circle of friends who bring meals and conversation for an hour a day or a family member who takes over the laundry and dishes for the first week.

This is not just a checklist of a few household tasks to take over but a precious gift allowing the mother to recover her strength and focus solely on her own recovery and the baby. *It takes a village, rooted in Christ, for that is where we find rest and renewal in this precious season with a fresh earthside babe.* [6]

New mothers need more than just self-help books, free meals, and less tasks to do. Postpartum mothers need a village – a community of friends, family, and perhaps a postpartum doula, who come together to give her support in a way that fits her needs while using their respective gifts, allowing her voice to be heard. [7]

I will say it again: you are chosen by God for this precious season of pregnancy, birth, and the days with a fresh babe, as well as those to come in motherhood. Steward this time well by learning about the importance of rest, the importance of community and your village, and the importance of caring for your whole mind, body, and spirit during this time.

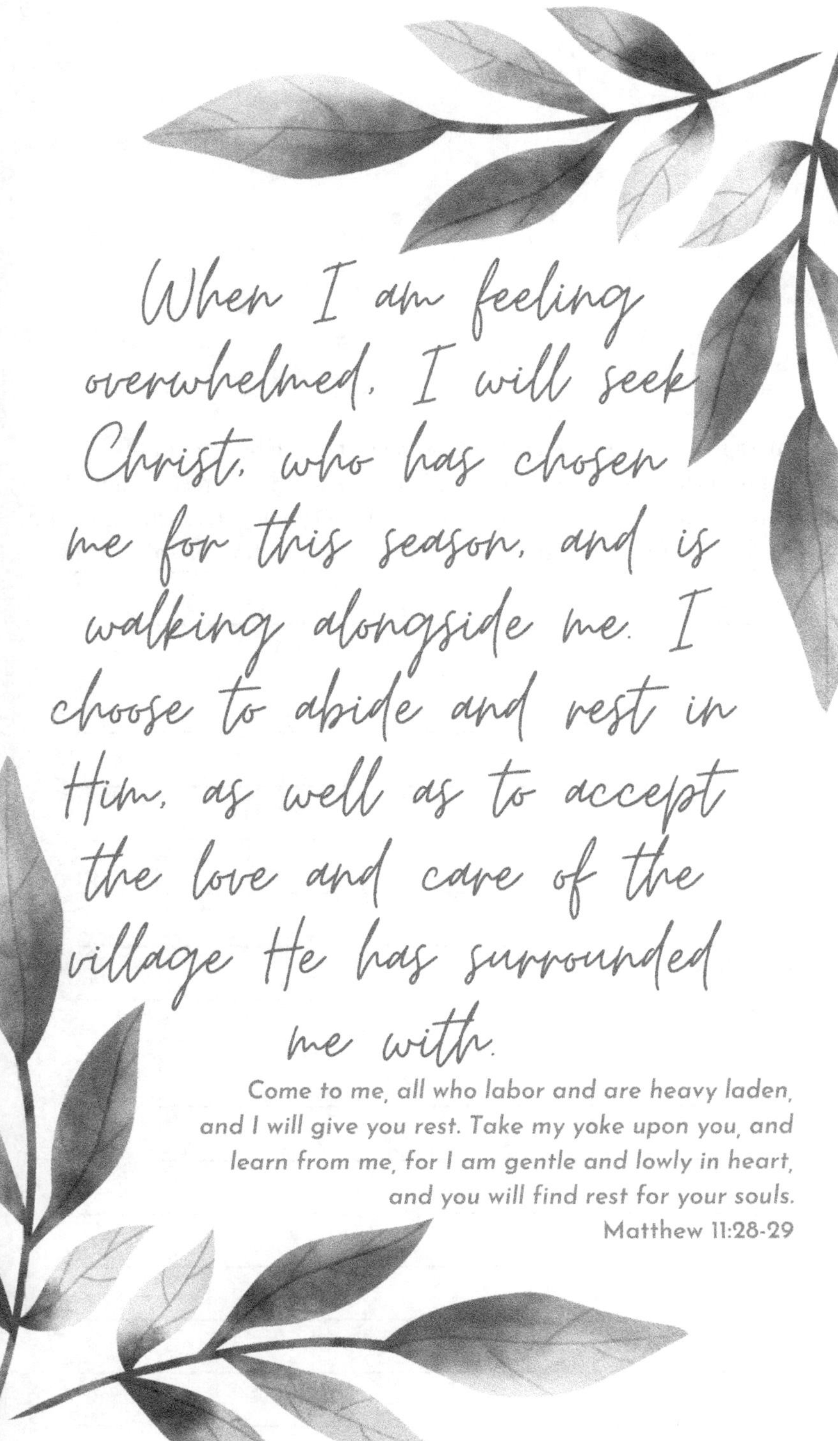
When I am feeling overwhelmed, I will seek Christ, who has chosen me for this season, and is walking alongside me. I choose to abide and rest in Him, as well as to accept the love and care of the village He has surrounded me with.

Come to me, all who labor and are heavy laden, and I will give you rest. Take my yoke upon you, and learn from me, for I am gentle and lowly in heart, and you will find rest for your souls.
Matthew 11:28-29

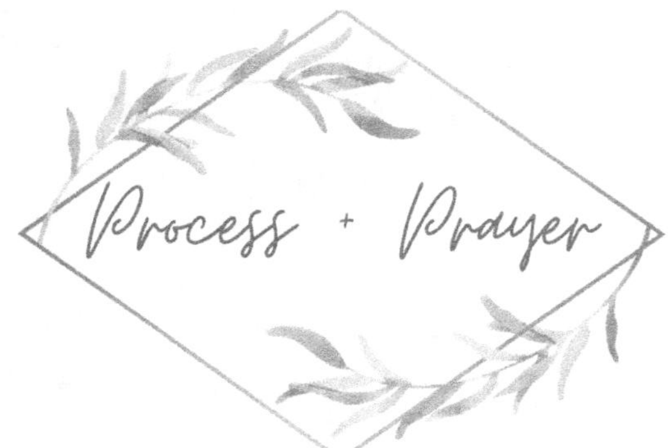

Take a few minutes to reflect on how being chosen by God for this season affects how you seek to steward your time, pursuing rest + renewal postpartum. Write a prayer to God, thanking Him for His sustenance and the community we have with other Christians, who come alongside.

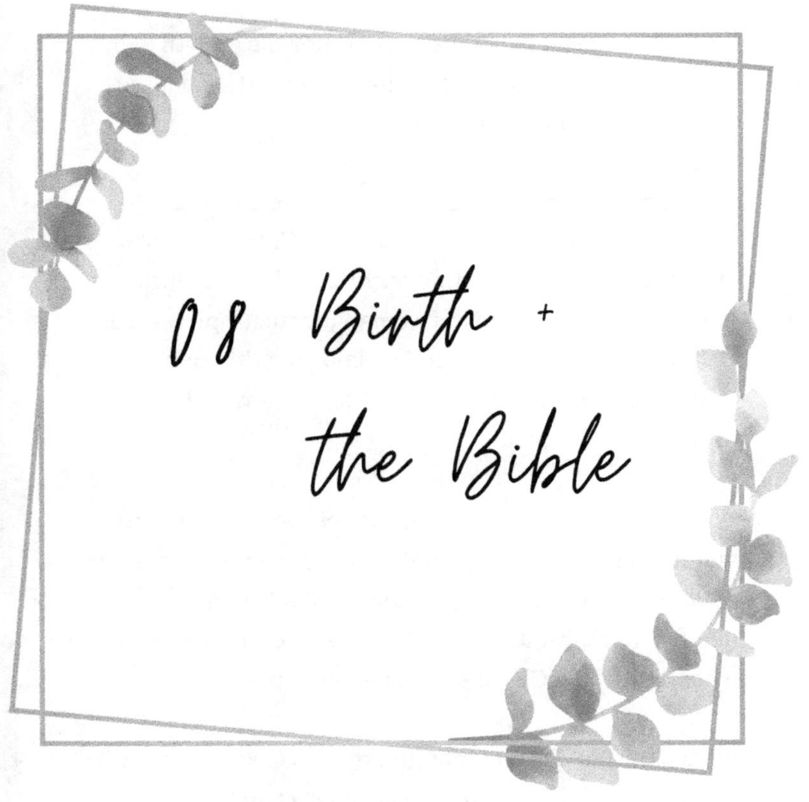

08 Birth + the Bible

Childbirth has existed since the first woman, Eve, gave birth. God designed birth, God values pregnancy, Jesus walks alongside you in pregnancy, and the gospel redeems and transforms pregnancy [1].

Our lives are proof of this, and as Christian women, we can honor our faith during labor in many ways.

One of the most important, perhaps for the growth of our faith, is by understanding the history of birth from the Bible, and through today [2].

In fact, an understanding of this arc in Scripture, completed by God made flesh in Jesus Christ, works to enhance our understanding of childbirth and makes us marvel at how God chose a woman for such a pivotal role in His story. He chose us, and by knowing this, our understanding of birth and the Bible is gloriously illuminated.

The verbiage used in Scripture which God speaks to us about labor and birth, should have a great pull in our view of labor. A consistent way God speaks to His chosen people, first the nation of Israel, and second, those of us whose faith is in Christ, is through metaphor.

In fact, the Old Testament often related God to giving birth to the nation Israel such as in Isaiah 42, and the New Testament related a spiritual rebirth by Jesus' work on the cross, in John 3.

With these examples in mind, *how does the way labor is discussed in Scripture affect how we view our part in birth and the greater biblical narrative today?*

Remember the premise surrounding Chosen; where we explore the intersection of birth and faith; Where we know in every fiber of our being that God called us individually, from our own mother's womb - He knew us by name, hair color, temperament, shoe size, and all.

If God went to such great lengths for us in the womb and today and tomorrow with the work of the Cross, Him who designed birth itself and chose us to be His vessels for new life, *why should we not look to Him to learn more of birth and take an active role in the process?*

In truth, much has changed in the way we view birth from biblical times until today, and we have much to learn. In fact, pregnancy and the act of labor itself isn't referenced explicitly in the Bible; Mostly it states that a woman became pregnant, then she had a child, and the story continues [3]. So much mystery of her experience and thoughts are not included. Scripture isn't dripping with instructions on childbirth, but it is teeming with metaphor and language surrounding childbirth and labor.

Indeed, There is still an aura of mystery surrounding childbirth - despite the technologies and advancements - so much is still unknown on the details, the when and how. Mystery is sustained, as well as the discomforts common in pregnancy and labor. What we cannot control is further put into a box in an attempt to reign in on the process, a man-made antidote to fear of God's design, and in this we limit ourselves.

Yet we do know that it was always a part of God's plan: if theology is the study of God, we can safely say that childbirth is in fact, theological, as it's a part of His design for us [4].

There is no way around it - childbirth is a fact of life; Childbirth matters for the future of God's chosen people and nation - in fact, childbirth matters for the future of humanity. It is woven into every story in the Bible, some more implicitly, others explicitly.

Birth history begins at Creation, continues through God's chosen people, and lasts today and tomorrow.

Looking at the nation of Israel, conversation around inheritance and the firstborn is precedent. Israelites believed and were told directly that their inheritance from God was the land of Canaan, which indeed became the nation of Israel --- knowing about this chosen land gave hope during years of wandering. This land could become their nation only if there were subsequent generations [5].

There is certainly a more specific birth history described in the Bible; it was common for midwives to manage prenatal and birth care for Hebrew mothers, and they practiced much like the nurse practitioners and midwives today [6].

In fact, two midwives in the Bible we know by name: Puah and Shiphrah. In Exodus 1:15-20 we find that they feared God and saved male Hebrew newborns, in direct opposition to Pharaoh's edict to kill baby boys at birth; Because of this, God honored them by giving the women families of their own.

In Genesis 30:3 an indirect reference of a woman being

supported in labor, as Rachel gives her servant to Jacob, to bear a child for her, stating that "she shall bear upon my knees." This phrasing indicates that she would aide her servant during labor by being the midwife, positioning for support [7]. For those familiar with birth work, the mother would be held upright and assisted in her balance, while allowing room for the baby to birth into the hands of the midwife, or assistance - in this case, Rachel.

Later, in Exodus 1:16 we read of delivery stools, to provide support for the mother in delivery. Typically these stools were made with hand grips, a back to lean against, and a crescent-shaped hole in the seat [8].

With these examples we can see that there was much freedom given during birth to what suited mom best; we also see this today in many practices, which support modern variations of delivery stools, birth balls, as well as additional forms of support available, such as professional doulas.

There is yet another verse from Galatians. It is quite obscure, and you'd almost miss the reference if you read it all together. Although not the most well-known verse about the value of life and an unborn child, it is important for a biblical understanding of birth, as it interprets your view of how Christ chooses you, and enriches your own faith and birth experiences.

Galatians 1:15-16 states, "But when God, *who had set me apart before I was born, and who called me by His grace,* was pleased to reveal His Son in me so that I might preach Him among the Gentiles, my immediate response was not to consult any human being." (emphasis mine)

The first part of this passage references a child in a mother's womb. This is from the letter Paul wrote to the churches in Galatia; it is a direct reference to what he knows of our origin and faith---that we are all set apart by God and we have all been called out by Him, given His grace, and known from before we were born.

We were known in our mothers wombs. Our babies in our wombs are also known intricately by God.

We were set apart, sanctified, chosen. The same goes for our children and every person you know.

And in knowing this, we also grow in our knowledge of and understanding of birth, from biblical times to today.

Chosen before birth, chosen for the season of birth, chosen by God. He doesn't choose you because of your birth plans, the amount of time you've spent studying birth, the number of times you've given birth, the method or way you give birth, or the number of births you have attended. He chooses you because He loves you, He created you, and He knows you [9].

In this, the season of pregnancy and birth is used to bend your heart toward Him, as He creates new life within you. And our response? To celebrate our part in God's design of birth - no matter the type of birth had.

Just as the lyrics state in "No Longer Slaves," which is based on Psalm 22:10; "From my mother's womb, You have chosen me, Love has called my name." [10]

In John 16:20-22, Jesus described a woman who endured

the pain of labor only to forget that pain in the joy of the arrival of her baby. In the same way, there is sorrow in this world, but when Jesus comes again, His children will forget that sorrow in light of their everlasting joy. (*See the affirmation for this chapter on more*)

Much has changed in the way we view birth from biblical times until today, and we have much to learn. There is still an aura of mystery surrounding childbirth - despite the technologies and advancements - so much is still unknown on the details, the when and how.

Mystery is sustained, as well as the discomforts common in pregnancy and labor.

What we cannot control is further put into a box in an attempt to reign in on the process, a man-made antidote to fear of God's design, and in this we limit ourselves.

Yet it's by this limit in which we actually cheapen the power of the gospel, the power of God's word for us. Because by understanding birth in the bible through the lens of a gift, a time which you are chosen for, you in turn alter your view from one of a burden, to one of a gift.

As Gloria Furman explains in an article for the Gospel Coalition, childbirth is evidence of God's mercy for us. He chose to give Adam and Eve the gift to multiply after sin, although they deserved death. Yet he chose life for us, as individuals, and he chose to invite us into the birth process, as how he created women. Life is a precious gift from a holy and just God [11].

Indeed, knowing we are chosen by God for this season

affects our understanding of birth through the lens of Scripture, and benefits us immensely today; By knowing this, we can be equipped in the labor to come to hold steadfast to our faith, no matter what happens. [12, 13]

For your identity as a mother is not in what happens in your labor; It is only found in Christ. He has already chosen you [14], and He continues to work in your story, just as He has throughout the Bible, and each day in your life. *Rest in these truths and watch as they enrich your own views of birth and faith!*

Your labor is not in vain [15]; God is with you, mama;

Know this truth, that you are, in fact, chosen.

Each contraction and pain brings us closer to meeting our answered prayer and fulfilled promise. This labor is not in vain. God is here with me, and my baby is almost here. I can do this, by Christ's strength!

A woman giving birth to a child has pain because her time has come, but when her baby is born, she forgets the anguish because of her joy that a child is born into the world

John 16:21

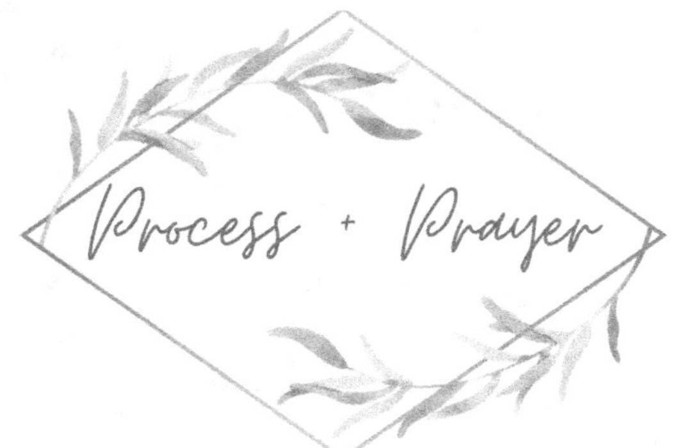

Take a few minutes to reflect on how being chosen by God for this season affects how you seek to understand birth in the Bible, as well as equips and strengthens you in labor. Write a prayer to God, thanking Him for the gift of Scripture, and for the gift of participating in His design of birth.

____

____

____

____

____

____

____

____

____

____

____

____

____

Acknowledgements

I've always read the acknowledgements in the dozens of books a year read, and wondered what I'd write in my own. So here we go.

This book wouldn't have even happened if I didn't sign up for hope*writers - of which, I am so grateful for, as it is such a life-giving gift. In fact, most of those I'd like to thank for this book, I met in hope*writers. It is truly the kindest place on the internet for writers.

For our next right thing hope*circle - linking arms with and cheering each other on, as our projects have morphed and taken shape, has been a privilege and a joy. Becky, Jen, Charity, Sarah, Rachel, Rachael, Melissa, Carly, Cathy, Trish, and more; I am grateful.

To the self-publishing and podcasting 101 hope*circles - thank you for answering my 20-questions-a-day on how to get started once I thought of each crazy idea - the less-than-2-weeks from in my head to in listeners' ears podcast, and the same time-frame for deciding on self-publishing the transcripts. Thank you for the accountability, and for being my biggest cheerleaders and sounding board of all the things.

To the Her View From Home writing team, thank you for welcoming me into your community, and for giving me the confidence I needed in writing by publishing my article on grief. I am grateful to always have that corner of the internet to turn to for learning about all the writing and social media and motherhood things.

Acknowledgements

To those who endorsed this book and backed up the message, while showing such grace, encouragement, and generosity in your words; thank you for being willing, and thank you for lending your voice to this project. I am humbled by your kind words.

To those who edited and gave constructive feedback on these words as they were articles, then podcast transcripts, then a one sheet and book proposal, then chapters; and to Kayla, who proofread these words; I am grateful for your work.

To my family, for supporting me, and caring for my boys in the fringe minutes so that I could catch up on edits and compiling these transcripts, thank you. Thank you for so much more than words can say here, for all the ways you've come alongside me and my boys as we've needed it.

To my two boys, who have taught me to seek joy in each moment, and have shown me such grace and joy in motherhood, It is because of the gift of your lives, and the experience of your births, that I began to write the blog posts, which turned into a book proposal, which turned into a podcast, which turned into this book - for I wouldn't even know of this gift of grace which childbirth is, nor seek to share it with others, if it weren't for y'all. Taylor and Travis, I am immeasurably grateful to be your mama.

To my blog readers, podcast listeners, email receivers, social media followers, and internet friends (and to you); thank you for showing up and being ready to listen and read whenever I muster up words to speak; I pray that these words are read as gifts to you, and I'm honored to share them with you.

Acknowledgements

These are words I wish I had at a time when I needed them, preparing for pregnancy/birth. Grateful to be able to serve you with them, and I pray they bless you and enrich your faith throughout this precious time - ultimately, pointing you to Christ.

To my church family and community group at OneLife; it's hard to explain how I felt such immense peace when I first set foot in the doors. Over and over I have witnessed firsthand how you relentlessly and persistently pursue Christ, while focusing on community, and stressing the importance of reading Scripture accurately and in context; This has brought me back to life as well as to tears when I allow myself to dwell on it, things of my faith I am re-learning. Especially following a season which was tragic yet is now marked with healing; Truly, I cannot adequately put to words how meaningful the community and friendships I've gained through our common thread of faith and belief in Jesus, have been. For this, I am grateful.

For Jesus, whose unrelenting pursuit of my heart and mind during my pregnancies and motherhood and life sparked a thought of this book into existence; because birth + faith are not compartmentalized, and if more Christian women knew these simple truths, fear would turn into awe, anxiety would turn into peace, pain would turn into glory; even stretch marks would be seen as grace; And how would this transform our lives, families, and communities for the better?!

Thank you, Jesus, for being born to us in order to redeem us: These words barely scratch the surface of how interwoven our personal experiences of birth and our understanding of

Acknowledgements

theology, the study of God, truly are.

It truly takes a village to birth a book (get it?!), and I can go on for fifty pages covering all of the fingerprints and prayers of others who have helped to shape this message, and form it into what you hold in your hands.

But since there is no space for that, I will end by stating that this isn't about me, or even those who have come alongside in this project; Because while a village is pivotal, the goal of this book is to ultimately point you to Christ in the season of pregnancy, birth, and birth work; For as stated in the dedication, these words barely scratch the surface of how interwoven our experiences of birth and understanding of theology, the study of God, truly are. Yet here they are, wrapped in book form, as a gift, just for you.

I pray these words meet you where you are and rejuvenate, refocus your sight on Jesus, during this time of preparation for birth.

Thank you, all. I am grateful.

Notes

CHAPTER 1

1. Newsom, K. "God is in the grief of unmet expectations" Her View From Home. https://www.herviewfromhome.com/god-is-in-the-grief-of-unmet-expectations/
2. Newsom, K. "My birth story: I gave birth in a car." Motherly. https://www.motherly.com/life/my-birth-story-i-gave-birth-in-a-car/
3. Smith, Aubry G. (2016) *Holy Labor: How Childbirth Shapes A Woman's Soul*. Kirkdale Press.
4. L'Engle, Madeline. *Walking on Water: Reflections on Faith and Art*, Convergent Books, 2016 Edition.
5. Freeman, Emily P. (2013) *A Million Little Ways: Uncover The Art You Were Made To Live*, Revell, Baker Publishing Group.
6. Newsom, K. See Reference #1.
7. Smith, Aubry G. See Reference #3.

CHAPTER 2

1. Newsom, K. "Dear Pregnant Mama, the Gospel Transforms Your Pregnancy" Christ-Centered Mama. https://www.christcenteredmama.com/dear-pregnant-mama-the-gospel-transforms-your-pregnancy/
2. "The Baby In Your Womb: God's Workmanship" Cold Waters to a Thirsty Soul.. 18 January 2015. https://www.coldwatertoathirstysoul.wordpress.com/2015/01/18/the-baby-in-your-womb-gods-workmanship/
3. "Baby's Heartbeat" *Just The Facts.* https:www.justthefacts.org/get-the-facts/babys-heartbeat/
4. Newsom, K. See Reference #1.
5. Kulick, Alexandra N. (2017) *Re:Birth: Pregnancy Restored.* CreateSpace Independent Publishing Platform.

CHAPTER 3

1. Epstein, Randi H. (2011) *Get Me Out: A History of Childibrth from the Garden of Eden to the Spem Bank*, W.W. Norton & Company.
2. Furman, Gloria. "10 Convictions About Labor and Birth from a Christian Worldview" The Gospel Coalition. 5 January 2016. https://www.thegospelcoalition.org/article/10-convictions-about-labor-and-birth-from-a-christian-worldview/
3. Bergmann, Claudia D. Bible Odyssey, People. "Pregnancy and Childbirth in the Hebrew Bible." https://www.bibleodyssey.org/en/people/related-articles/pregnancy-and-childbirth-in-the-hebrew-bible
4. Furman, Gloria. See Reference#2.
5. Stovel, Beth M. (2012) "The Birthing Spirit, the Childbearing God: Metaphors of Motherhood and their Place in Christian Discipleship" Priscilla Press (Vol 26, No 4) https://www.cbeinternational.org/sites/default/files/Birthing_Stovell.pdf

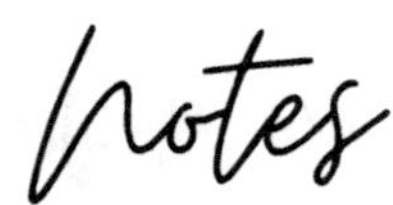

Notes

CHAPTER 4

1. Martin, Chelsea. 2015 September 25. "The Hope Of Birthing For His Glory" Surrender Birth. https://www.surrenderbirth.com
2. "Birth Affirmations Help Reduce Stress And Build Confidence" https://www.mygentleborn.com/en/birth-affirmations-reduce-stress/

CHAPTER 5

1. L'Engle, Madeline. *Walking on Water: Reflections on Faith and Art*, Convergent Books, 2016 Edition.
2. Brown, Brene. 2017. *Rising Strong: How the Ability to Reset Transforms the Way We Live, Love, Parent, and Lead*. Random House Trade Paperbacks.
3. Estoria, Arielle. opening spoken word performance at the 2019 hope*writers conference in Charlotte, NC.
4. Estoria, Arielle. See Reference #3.
5. Newsom, K. 18 Feburary 2020. "Episode 05 // How Knowing We Are Chosen Prompts Us To Write And Share Our Stories Of Birth" Simple Natural Mama. https://www.simplenaturalmama.com/2020/02/18/episode-05-how-knowing-we-are-chosen-prompts-us-to-write-and-share-our-stories-of-birth/
6. Newsom, K. 13 Februray 2020. "Faith Is Like A Doula" Simple Natural Mama. https://www.simplenaturalmama.com/2020/02/13/faith-is-like-a-doula/

CHAPTER 6

1. Villines, Zawn. 12 January 2020. "What are the miscarriage rates by week?" Medical News Today. https://www.medicalnewstoday./com/articles/322634#pregnancy-loss-rates-by-week
2. Newsom, K. "God is in the grief of unmet expectations" Her View From Home. https://www.herviewfromhome.com/god-is-in-the-grief-of-unmet-expectations/
3. Starr, Michelle. 1 August 2018. "New Research Shows Most Human Pregnancies End In Miscarriage" Science Altert, Humans. https://www.sciencealert.com/meta-analysis-finds-majority-of-human-pregnancies-end-in-miscarriage-biorxiv/amp
4. Newsom, K. "When Birth Didn't Go As Planned." 17 October 2019. Christ-Centered Mama. https://www.christcenteredmama.com/when-birth-didnt-go-as-planned/
5. Newsom, K. "What You Need To Know About Pregnancy And Infant Loss Awareness Day." 15 October 2019. Simple Natural Mama. https://www.simplenaturalmama.com/2019/10/15/what-you-need-to-know-about-pregnancy-and-infant-loss-awareness-day/

Notes

CHAPTER 7

1. Newsom, K. "Self-Care in the Postpartum Period" Jen Roland, Self-Care For The Christian Woman series. https://www.jenroland.com.
2. Postpartum Doula Certification. Madriella Doula Network. Accessed 2019.
3. Newsom, K. See Reference #1.
4. "We Were Made For Community" BLOG for the NIV New International Version Bible. https://www.thenivbible.com/we-were-made-for-community
5. Goldberg, Joel. "It Takes A Village To Determine The Origins Of An African Proverb." 30 July 2016. https://www.NPR.org/goatsandsoda/2016/07/30/487925796/it-takes-a-village-to-determine-the-origins-of-an-african-proverb/
6. Newsom, K. 2019 September 13. "Postpartum Mothers Need A Village, And Here's Why" Simple Natural Mama, https://www.simplenaturalmama.com/2019/09/13/postpartum-mothers-need-a-village-and-heres-why/
7. Newsom, K. See Reference #1.

CHAPTER 8

1. Newsom, K. 2019 April 21. "Dear Pregnant Mama, the Gospel Transforms Your Pregnancy." Christ-Centered Mama. https://www.christcenteredmama.com/dear-pregnant-mama-the-gospel-transforms-your-pregnancy/
2. Smith, Carol. (2012) Women of the Bible: A Visual Guide To Their Lives, Loves & Legacy. Illustrated Bible Handbook Series. Barbour Publishing, Inc.
3. Smith, Carol. See Reference #2.
4. Smith, Aubry G. (2016) *Holy Labor: How Childbirth Shapes A Woman's Soul.* Kirkdale Press.
5. Smith, Carol. See Reference #2.
6. Smith, Carol. See Reference #2.
7. Smith, Carol. See Reference #2
8. Smith, Carol. See Reference #2.
9. Myers, Michelle. (2018) *100 she works HIS way Devotionals for the Working Woman.* Myers Cross Training.
10. Bethel Music. "No Longer Slaves" We Will Not Be Shaken, 2015, Track Number 4, https://www.bethelmusic.com
11. Furman, Gloria. "10 Convictions About Labor and Birth from a Christian Worldview." The Gospel Coalition. 5 January 2016, https://www.thegospelcoalition.org/article/10-convictions-about-labor-and-birth-from-a-christian-worldview/
12. Newsom, K. 10 September 2019. "10 Biblical Affirmation Cards For Labor" Simple Natural Mama. https://www.simplenaturalmama.com/
13. Newsom, K. 4 February 2020. "Episode 03 // How Being Chosen Prompts Us To Better Understand And Prepare For Childbirth" Simple Natural Mama. https://www.simplenaturalmama.com/
14. Myers, Michelle. (2018) *100 she works HIS way Devotionals for the Working Woman.* Myers Cross Training.
15. The Porter's Gate. "Your Labor Is Not In Vain." Work Songs: The Porter's Gate Worship Project Vol 1, The Fuel Music, 2017, Track Number 13, https://www.theportersgate.com

Scripture Index

*The following passages are directly or indirectly referenced
in the corresponding chapters:*

Scripture Index

*The following passages are directly or indirectly referenced
in the corresponding chapters:*

About the Author

Katherine Leigh is a writer, podcast host, birth and postpartum doula, and childbirth educator, who lives in the gulf coast of Texas with her family. As a work-at-home mom to her two young boys, she spends her days as a writing tutor for college students, writing for publication, and creating birth and postpartum resources for new moms (including courses!). She writes on her website, *Simple Natural Mama*, for the Christian mom who is simple and natural minded.

Her writing has also appeared in *The Joyful Life Magazine*, *Her View From Home*, *Motherly*, *Mama Natural*, *Christ-Centered Mama*, and for the *Grounded Conferences Ministry*.

You can find her at *www.simplenaturalmama.com*, on Facebook as *Simple Natural Mama*, or on Instagram at *@katherineleighwrites*

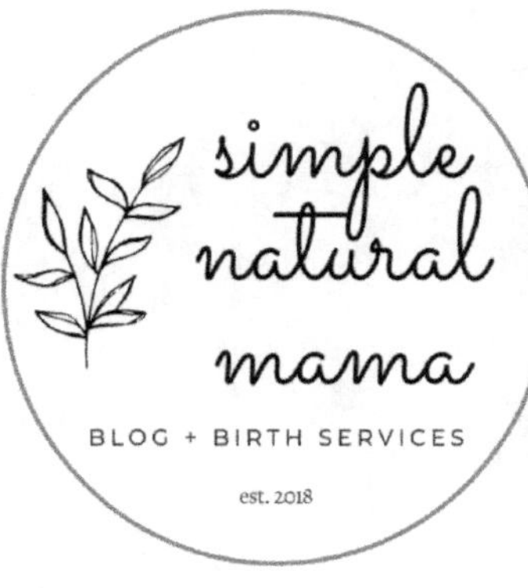

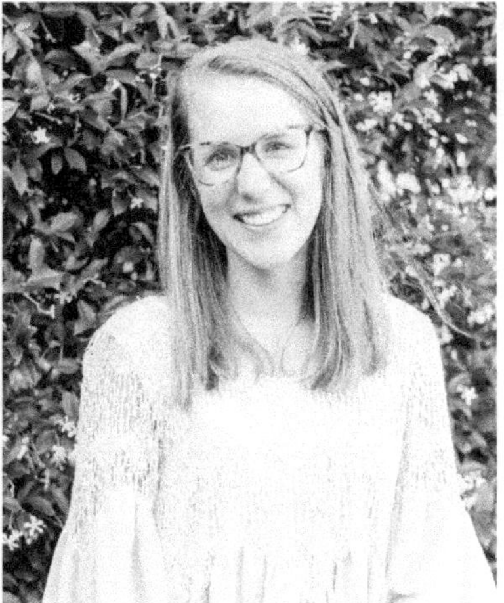

Gifts For You!

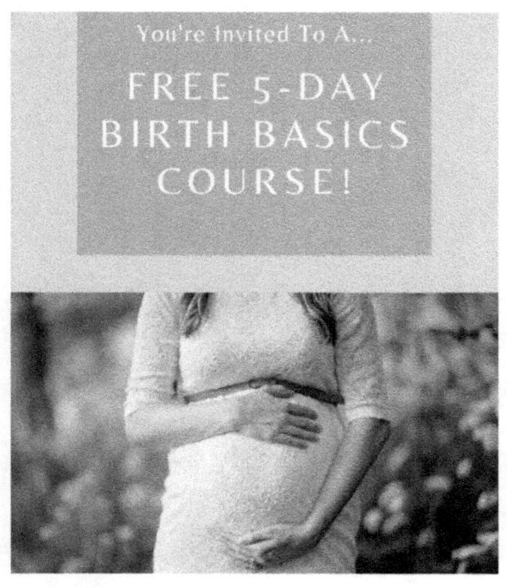

Jumpstart Your Birth Preparation
With A FREE 5-Day Course!

Does birth seem overwhelming and like a mystery to you?

Are you interested in learning more of the birth process and comfort measures?

Would you like a quick primer on what to expect and suggestions on how to prepare, from the help of a doula?

If you answered yes to these questions, sign up for this 5-day email course, delivered straight to your inbox!

Just head to www.simplenaturalmama.com and click on *Education Services* to get started!

Gifts For You!

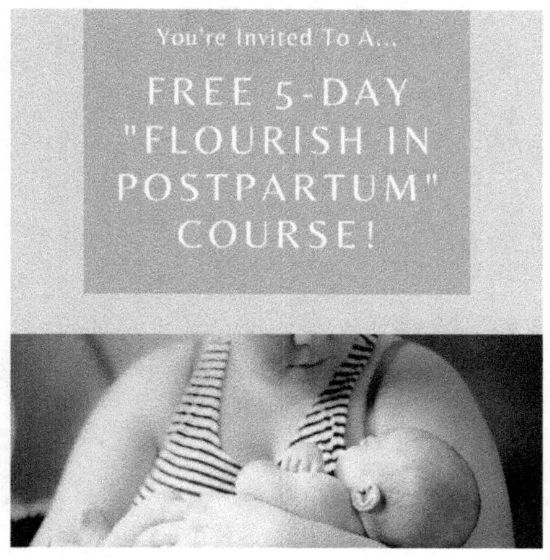

Feel Prepared For Life Postpartum
With A FREE 5-Day Course!

Does postpartum - life with a newborn - seem overwhelming and like a mystery to you?

Are you interested in learning more of the changes to your mind and body postpartum?

Would you like a quick primer on what to expect and suggestions on how to prepare, from the help of a postpartum doula?

If you answered yes to these questions, sign up for this 5-day email course, delivered straight to your inbox!

Just head to www.simplenaturalmama.com and click on *Education Services* to get started!

Gifts For You!

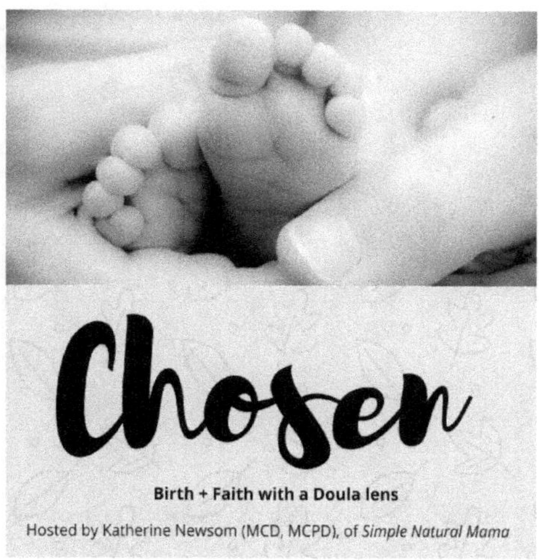

Do you prefer audio content, instead?

Are you an expecting mother or birth worker who is also a woman of God, and wants to find a biblical perspective on birth?

Are you interested in learning about birth from someone who actually works in the birth industry, in this current generation?

Are you simply curious of learning more about pregnancy and birth from a faith-based perspective, whether it's for your own growth or to be able to better relate to your mama friends?

I've hosted the *Chosen: Birth + Faith With A Doula Lens* podcast just for you.

Just head to www.simplenaturalmama.com and click on *Podcast* to find where to listen, as well as additional supplemental materials. You can also search *Chosen: Birth + Faith Through A Doula Lens* on your favorite podcast player, at anytime!

Note: Per the copyright page, this book was compiled based on the first season of the Chosen podcast, with changes and additions. Rather than an audiobook version, why not listen to the original podcast which this book came from?

Gifts For You!

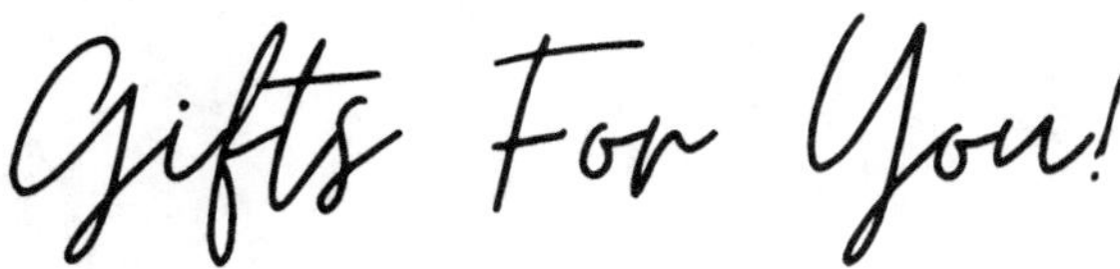

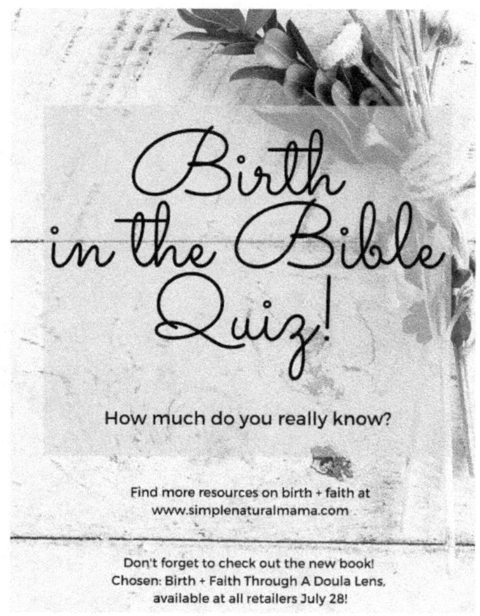

How much do you really know about birth in the Bible?

Do you want to take your faith and knowledge of birth a step further, with practical Bible trivia?

How much do you know about the women, midwives, and narratives concerning birth in the Bible, anyway?

Take the quiz to find out!

There are a total of 20 questions, scripture references, and 4 results, based on your knowledge! You are welcome tp print out the document and share with your friends, also!

Just head to www.simplenaturalmama.com, click on the above photo, and enter your information to automatically download the PDF.